80E-395

Visual Handicaps and Learning

A Developmental Approach

Natalie C. Barraga

University of Texas at Austin

Wadsworth Publishing Company, Inc.
Belmont, California

Wadsworth Series in Special Education

Series Editor: Eli M. Bower
University of California, Berkeley

Deafness and Learning: A Psychosocial Approach
Hans G. Furth
The Catholic University of America

The Exceptional Child: A Primer
Lita Linzer Schwartz
The Pennsylvania State University, Ogontz Campus

Visual Handicaps and Learning: A Developmental Approach
Natalie Barraga
University of Texas at Austin

ISBN 0–534–00434–2

L. C. Cat. Card No. 75–27715

Printed in the United States of America

1 2 3 4 5 6 7 8 9 10—80 79 78 77 76

Foreword

There is little doubt that the loss of sight presents a great ego difficulty for the human animal. Most adults, given the unhappy (and theoretical) choice of reducing their five senses to four, would not be without sight. Life is intimately tied to vision, yet thousands of our fellow beings live in what John Milton described as "the ever enduring dark."

The loss of sight is traumatic in both perception and reality. Our world is made up of symbols of which words, images, and pictures are major vehicles. The full implications of loss of vision are seldom understood by the seeing. Several years ago college students volunteering for work with children at the School for the Blind in Berkeley were asked to spend a day living at the school in a "blinded" state. When they arrived in the morning, they were blindfolded. As they went about their duties and tasks of the day, they were videotaped. Later they were shown videotapes of their blindfolded day. All saw themselves as becoming more and more psychologically constricted—head down, posture bent and curled, and walk tentative. Some had so "aged" physically by the end of the day that they could not recognize themselves.

The air, water, and earth that surround us make up the personal and moving space in which we live. This space is a product of our vision. When this space cannot be predicted or utilized with confidence the organism falters.

So the education of children with vision problems involves not only a problem of encoding and decoding symbols but how the ego relates to self and environment. Dr. Barraga has brought excellent professional experience and high personal concern to bear on this complex problem—the growth and learning of children with vision problems. Readers will better understand the problems of blind and partially sighted children as well as the gift and miracle of the eye and the brain.

Eli M. Bower
Berkeley, California

Preface

Historical documents and literature throughout the ages have expressed a concern about impairments in sensory organs, especially in the eye. Philosophers have theorized that the eye was a mystical organ related to the soul; some have supported legal sanctions for destruction of those without sight; others have advocated veneration and worship of blind persons; while a few have actually suggested isolated care as a benevolent societal attitude. Not until the seventeenth century was consideration given to the idea of education. Even then, the major concern for hundreds of years was one of training for service to society. The general public today considers vision the most prized of all the senses. Superstitions and emotionally laden attitudes are still associated with visual impairment or with the concept of blindness; those who are able to learn and succeed without sight are a source of amazement to many.

The person *becomes* his problem, whether it is no more than a minor impairment or a total lack of visual functioning. Misconceptions and distortions have hindered educators in their attempts to present more realistic ideas about children with visual impairments. Acceptance and integration into educational settings on the same terms as any children who have physical or other differences is an ideal toward which parents and educators are still striving.

To understand the areas of limitations related to visual impairments, we must think objectively about the role of vision in learning and plan interventions appropriate to the nature and degree of the limitations, so that all dimensions of development are permitted to expand concurrently in relation to what a child is capable of learning and doing. Emphasizing what capacities a child has, how he can develop, and what guidance will facilitate optimal functioning should be the primary approach. To redirect thinking toward this goal, attention focused on causes or medical diagnoses of eye conditions, which stress visual damage and incapacity, should be shifted toward undamaged organs and the potential for development and learning through alternative senses and processes.

The discussions in this text are addressed to special education students, vision and/or eye specialists, and any other interested person who may wish to read them. A new way of thinking about individuals with visual impairments will be presented in the hope that limitations in visual capacity will come to be viewed from a total perspective of human development, and also that potential for learning to be a participating member of a "seeing world" may be realized.

Although frequent reference will be made to the possible effects of visual handicaps on self-concept, personality characteristics, and social interactions, the primary thrust will be on developmental processes and facilitating learning. Discussions will center on behavioral responses—affective, psychomotor, and cognitive dimensions as influenced by the kind and extent of the visual handicap.

Developmental and learning processes will be presented from a descriptive and functional frame of reference rather than as generalized characteristics, factual data, or statistical information relying heavily on measurement criteria. Some ideas discussed in the text are based on personal experiences of many years; others have emerged through study, observation, and research. As the mother of a child visually handicapped from birth, a teacher of children for many years, and more recently as a teacher educator, my approach has been formed through translating theory into practice. From these roles I have developed a deep philosophy that includes a firm belief that neither measurements, labels, materials, equipment, nor legislation is as important as the personal factors in human beings—both teachers and students—as they relate to or influence development and learning. Regardless of what labels may be applied, the educator's major concern must be to develop to the fullest each child's potential for learning.

The vignettes presented in Chapter 1 are purely fictional and do not describe any real persons known to me through personal experience or from reading actual case histories. The children depicted represent the variability in severity of visual impairments and the range and diversity of the influence on development and learning. Children similar to those portrayed are likely to be found in almost any community or school setting. Description of a multi-impaired, visually handicapped child is omitted purposely because there is no representative example. Frequent reference to the children described in the vignettes is for the sole purpose of illustrating ideas and should not be associated with any real person.

Chapter 2 examines the problem of the multiplicity of descriptive terms, making an appeal for the adoption of appropriate terminology in an attempt to substitute stability of thought for stereotypic notions. Because environmentally influenced development and learning in all children begin immediately at birth, Chapters 3 and 4 identify the concerns of the earliest years of life and present a theoretical basis for evaluating developmental patterns reflected in learning behavior. Chapter 5 addresses the problem of visually handicapped children who have additional impairments that disrupt emotional and physical development and may limit markedly the potential for mental development.

Chapters 6 and 7 continue the basic developmental theme, identifying and analyzing the processes and means for cognitive development and academic learning. The issue of testing and other evaluative approaches to intellectual and personal functioning is explored in Chapter 8. The culmination of development and learning in achieving the goals of independent living and vocational success is considered in Chapter 9, prior to offering final suggestions in Chapter 10 for further translating knowledge into dynamic action.

Because these ideas have been fostered by many persons and evolved out of a wide variety of literary sources, documentation of references is more often general than specific. When appropriate, the reader is directed to specific references to undertake in-depth study.

The author assumes full responsibility for inaccuracies, provocative controversy, and limitations in discussions. Grateful appreciation is expressed to all of those children, teachers, students, and colleagues who have had a part in generating and shaping these thoughts through the years. I am indebted also to two graduate students, Jan Ozias and Judy Holt, who took time to read the manuscript and make critical suggestions.

Contents

Contents

1

To See or Not to See

The commonalities among children who have visual impairments are few and the differences are many. Some are totally blind from birth or become blind shortly thereafter. Many more have serious structural or pathological conditions of the eye at birth but are still able to function *visually* in an adequate manner throughout their lives. A few have medical conditions that become progressively serious until total blindness occurs at some time during the school years. In other cases, an accident may be responsible for sudden blindness in some children. As a means of emphasizing the differences among children and youth identified as visually handicapped, the following vignettes depict several typical children who have visual impairments.

Carl

As the counselor for visually handicapped and the young student of special education who was accompanying her approached the door, they heard a little boy say, "I hear somebody coming," and his mother responded with, "Thank you, I'll be there." The student looked at the counselor with a puzzled expression, since she had understood that they were going to see a totally blind child three-and-a-half years old. She wondered how he knew they were coming to his house.

As soon as the counselor spoke, Carl squealed her name and opened the door to grab her in a big hug just as the mother arrived. The student was introduced as the counselor's friend, and by the time they had entered and sat down, Carl was asking the young girl one question after another, as if she were already his friend, too.

Events of the past few moments had shattered the student's preconceived notions of blindness. She became so enchanted with Carl that all anxieties seemed to flow away as she sat quietly, watching and listening. She began to realize how much there was to learn by observing Carl as he moved about, played with his toys, and interacted with the adults. He was totally blind, but this fact was forgotten as soon as the mother and the counselor began a conversation. They responded to Carl's questions or interacted with him occasionally, when he was not totally absorbed in his own play. At times he would seek contact by approaching one of them or calling a name to determine whether they were still nearby.

In many ways, Carl seemed much like any other child of three-and-a-half, as he talked to himself, then to his toys, and at times to one of the adults. Other children might look for a smile or a wave of the hand for assurance or to maintain contact, but Carl frequently sought verbal interactions.

Although the student had not expected to see a child who would be moving from place to place so freely, she noted that when Carl moved he seemed to move to a voice; and that as he moved away from the voice, he was able to avoid chairs and other objects in the room just as if he could see them. When he was near another person, Carl would usually touch the person or the chair to maintain some bodily contact as he talked or questioned. Sometimes he asked for help in playing or for assistance in finding a particular toy; frequently Carl's mother described verbally where he would find the toy or instructed him that he could look in a particular place in his room for what he wanted. Encouraged and reassured by his mother, Carl searched with his hands until he found things and continued with his play; or he went to another room and came back with the object he wanted. If he left the room, he put out his hands to verify the location of doorways; he used his feet also to help him find toys that he thought were located in a general area.

During the visit, the student was somewhat surprised to hear the mother ask Carl to bring things to her, to take objects to the counselor, or to tell the visitors something about what he was doing. She even let him go outside by himself to ride his tricycle, after reminding him to ride only to the end of the sidewalk and then back to the front steps.

By the time she found herself outside with the counselor after cheerful goodbyes, the student's thoughts were going in all directions. She had so many questions: Are all three-year-old, totally blind children like Carl? Do all mothers relate to their blind children as Carl's mother did? How did he know to avoid a chair or to stop before he bumped into the door? Did he listen for cues that he couldn't see?

Continuing to reflect on the visit, she began to recall from her observations ways in which Carl differed from sighted three-year-old children. As he played or moved around, he seemed to hold his head down rather than up, unless reminded, and he made more than the usual amount of noise as he handled his toys and played with them, sometimes using them simply for the purpose of making a sound. Were all blind children so noisy in their play? She recalled also that if the conversation stopped and the room was very quiet, Carl would usually be the first one to say something, to ask a question, or to find some way to interact with one of the adults. Did she just imagine this or was it really so? Another thing seemed different—Carl frequently used his toys differently from other children's play, and not always for the purposes for which they were intended. He seemed to change often from one toy to another and to misplace his toys, at which time he moved to the adults to be a part of the group. What were the reasons for these differences?

Looking back over the total experience, the student had a good feeling, although she still felt much confusion and was unable to resolve all of her questions. Nevertheless, she recognized that some of her misconceptions were gone and that she would be quite comfortable with other blind children she might encounter.

Not all young blind children are like Carl, nor are all mothers like his mother in their attitudes and interactions with their children. Neither are all children who have visual handicaps totally blind, as you can see from the following description of another child, who was born with a severe visual impairment but was not totally blind.

Lucy

At the age of two, Lucy was still a puzzle to her parents; they had many conflicting thoughts about her. At the most unexpected moments she appeared to reach out toward things as if she could see them, and at other times she seemed not to be able to see at all. What had the doctor said when she was born? "Something is wrong with her eyes and we don't know how much she is going to be able to see, or whether she is going to see anything at all; we will just have to wait until she is older." Oh, yes, the doctor had said something else: "There is nothing medically we can do to help her, and I don't know anything to tell you to do." Fortunately for Lucy, her parents wanted a baby very much, and although they were confused and upset, she was so cuddly and lovable that they found it possible much of the time to think of her as they would have thought of any other baby.

Her parents gave her lots of love, they took her with them wherever they could, and the mother always watched for signs that Lucy *could* see. When she was a few weeks old, they noticed that she repeatedly turned her head when a light was turned on in the room and that she turned toward a window when being held. Was it possible that she could see the light? Several months later, when Lucy was enjoying being played with, she had tried to reach out toward a person's face, although she never followed her mother around the room with her eyes, and often her eyes seemed to move as if she had little control of them. At six months, when Lucy could sit up alone, she would often reach toward the soap in the bath water or extend an arm in the direction of her feet when being dressed. Surely these actions were indications that she was seeing something. At the age of one year, Lucy would pick up objects or toys and move them back and forth in front of her eyes, holding them very close to her face.

If she dropped or lost something she was playing with, she never seemed to be able to find it easily, and would either cry or "feel around" as if she could not see at all. Crawling, standing, and walking posed no real problems, although she was a bit hesitant to move very far and seldom directed her body purposively, except within a very limited area.

Despite their doubts, confusions, and many questions, Lucy's parents began to be very hopeful that she would be able to see after all. They played games with her trying to get her to focus on objects, to get her to find things, and they showed her everything possible in the house and outside. Soon they developed the habit of calling her attention to interesting things by saying, "Look, Lucy," and helping her direct her gaze toward the object. When only about eighteen months old, Lucy looked up at the moon one night and said, "Light." This was strange behavior for a child who could hardly see the food on her plate and who seemed always to be reaching for things by grasping not far enough or too far to the right or left, frequently knocking the object to the floor in her efforts.

By the time she was two-and-a-half, Lucy was grabbing for her clothes and trying to help put them on, especially if they were bright colors. Her mother also began to note that Lucy responded differently when colors were bright or there was good contrast between color and the background. As she sat in her mother's lap listening to stories, Lucy would clutch the book and pull it close to her face. Her mother would talk to her about what was in the pictures, and soon Lucy began to look for pictures in her books.

At the age of three, she began to look voluntarily at magazines she found in the house, and she showed much more interest in exploring. The parents talked to many specialists and were encouraged to continue to play "seeing games" with her, to invite her to look closely and carefully, and to assist her in seeing things or in moving her closer in order for her to be able to see better. By the time she was four, Lucy had begun to show interest in making marks with crayons, although she used them differently than other children did. Her pictures were not so much imitations of people or things as they were marks with many colors. She did seem to enjoy the experience of drawing and painting, just as other children of her age did.

In nursery school, Lucy could move from one piece of playground equipment to another and take her turns with other children, although there were many other tasks that she was not learning as readily or as easily as children who had no visual problem. For example, she might approach the swing without any indication that she could see that a child was swinging toward her; she often tripped over things directly in front of her, but could move several feet directly ahead to a dominantly visible object that she wanted.

As the time for her to begin elementary school came closer, her parents still had many questions about how much Lucy could see, how safe she was in certain situations, and what should be expected of her. Despite these uncertainties, her parents realized that Lucy had progressed a great deal in learning to be much more accurate in her use of vision; certainly she was far more interested in looking at things now than she had been in her earlier years. What would be the final result? Would Lucy be able to do her schoolwork? Would she learn to read by using the visual materials used by the other children, or would she have to learn to use braille?

Many severely visually handicapped children present a similar picture, and there are often few definitive answers. The prospects for such a child's future remain somewhat unclear; the child may behave sometimes as a seeing child and at other times as a child who cannot see at all. Parents, educators, and vision specialists can make few conclusive statements or predictions. Nevertheless, one possibility is evident—a child who demonstrates an ability to see may be able to learn to function more efficient visually. Certainly no child who can see to do the things that Lucy has been described as doing could be considered a "blind" child, even though this term was once used to describe her. As Lucy develops, there will continue to be many unanswered questions and many indecisions, but for the moment, Lucy is a child who sees and has already learned to explore her world visually and to find her place in relation to her little friends who have much better vision. With continued improvement, the prospect for Lucy's future may be more hopeful than for the child to be described next.

Dora

For the past ten years, Dora's parents had given little thought to what the doctor had told them when Dora was a baby—that he was not sure how healthy her eyes were, and although she probably would be fine and see perfectly for some years, the time might come when she would begin to lose her vision. The specialist had prescribed glasses for her when she was four. In the second grade, because Dora was having trouble keeping up in school, she had received assistance from a teacher specially trained to work with visually handicapped children.

Just today when they had taken her for an examination, Dora's parents had learned that she was losing her vision rapidly and *could be* totally blind in a few months. The shock was almost too much for them and they worried about whether or not to tell Dora. What would it do to her life if she knew? How would she feel? How would her friends react—would they still play with her? Why did it have to come now when she was still such a little girl? Would they even be able to discuss it with her without hurting and frightening her more?

Although the doctor had offered to explain the condition to Dora, her parents had rejected that idea, feeling that they could do it more gently. At first they thought about talking to Dora's teacher, but they decided that he would probably suggest getting help from counselors who work with blind people, and they weren't ready to think about Dora's being blind—not yet, anyway. Finally they realized that they *had* to talk with Dora, so they invited her to go for a drive.

"Dora, there is something we need to talk with you about," began her mother. The father said falteringly, "The doctor says that your eyes are not doing as well as they have been, and you seem to be losing some of your vision." Dora astounded them by her response. "Oh, I know that—I've known it for a long time, and I wondered when you were going to get around to talking about it! I asked my teacher about it when I knew I couldn't see so well any more, and he said not to worry about it. He gave me a magnifier and I can still read and do all my schoolwork."

Dora's mother wanted to take her in her arms and tell her how sorry she was, but she couldn't bring herself to do it because she knew that Dora would realize how sad she felt. As she was fumbling for something consoling to say to her daughter, the child continued, "The kids all help me, too, and when I drop something that I can't find, they tell me where it is until I get close enough to see it; that doesn't bother me since I never could see some things if the sun was shining or the light was too bright or if they were too far away. My friends have helped me before so they won't mind helping me even more."

As Dora continued to talk, her mother thought how much wiser than her years she sounded. "Ever since I noticed that I couldn't see as well, I've been practicing—sometimes I close my eyes and I try walking around by myself and you what? By just listening really well, I can tell a lot about what's going on and where the kids are and everything. When I have my eyes closed, I try to think about how things look, the way to get places, and I'll just keep on doing that when I can't see any more." The parents could find little to say, so they remained quiet and Dora kept talking. "Mother and Daddy, I think you should go and talk to my teacher. He'll help you understand things a lot better than you do now. He says I may still be able to read for a long time, because with a magnifier I can make the letters bigger and I already know what the words look like, and so I don't have to see them too clearly to tell what they are. And besides, when I can't see them well enough to read any more, my teacher's going to start letting me read with my fingers—you know, braille, like some of the other kids do. It's not so hard. Sometimes I get awfully tired when I try to read for too long or when I try to look too hard at things. My teacher says that when I learn braille, I'll be able to read with my eyes until I get tired and then read braille while I rest. And, do you know what? When I close my eyes and pick up things and feel them, I can already tell what they are."

When the parents were finally able to overcome their astonishment enough to relax and speak to their daughter, they told her how happy they were that she understood so well. In addition, they told Dora that she had explained much about her school work that they had not known before. They reminded her that there would be times when she would need to ask other people to help her, and that she must be much more careful about crossing streets and doing a lot of things that she had learned to do quite well, because if she didn't think about safety factors, she might get hurt. The parents tried very hard not to let Dora know their true feelings and great fears, because they knew it would only make it more difficult for their little daughter. They would try to be there to help her when she needed it and to comfort her when she had moments of frustration and impatience. But they realized that with a spirit like Dora's, somehow they, too, could accept the future.

Later that evening when they were alone, Dora's parents were able to think rationally. They realized that Dora had never been just like other children as far as her vision was concerned. She had used what sight she had and apparently hadn't worried about what she didn't have. Adjusting to a gradual loss in vision wasn't the same for her as it would have been for them. If she could take this in her stride and modify her thinking in such a positive way, they could stop feeling sad for her. It wasn't as if it were a sudden thing and there weren't time to plan, such as occurred in the following case.

Keith

Keith's father sat alone in the dark trying to think. It had been two weeks since the accident, and he could still hear the sound of the explosion and remember his dash down the stairs to the basement, in fearful panic of what might have happened to his son. When he had heard the boy scream, he recalled thinking, "Thank God, he's alive." Now his feelings were indescribable and his thoughts were so confused. The doctor had tried to be gentle when he had said, "Your son will live, but he will never see again." He recalled feeling that in the same moment, the doctor had assured life but had implied death.

If he could just turn back time, he would never have given twelve-year-old Keith that chemistry set. He felt responsible for his son's being blinded. Even his wife kept telling him it wasn't his fault—accidents happen. He knew he had to stop thinking about himself and start planning how he could help Keith adjust to a whole new way of living. He lay back in his chair and tried to interrupt his unhappy train of thought; he tried to conceive of all the hobbies and games that a boy could do without seeing. Maybe the counselor who had come to see them had had a good idea—that he could put on a blindfold and work with Keith. In fact, he would be learning something himself while he helped his son.

Soon his thoughts turned to all the things father and son used to do together, and it occurred to him that there was a way to alter most of their activities by using a little ingenuity and a lot of patience. They could still play ball—he'd roll it on the ground so Keith would hear it coming, and he could hit grounders. They could still go for walks and explore—he'd teach him how to recognize things with his hands so that Keith could still select rocks and leaves and other natural objects for his collections. Fishing would be just as much fun—maybe even more. After all, you feel the pole move before you see the cork go under when there is a bite.

The father sat upright in his chair as if startled by something. He had just remembered—school. How would Keith manage that? What was it the counselor had said about a special teacher who would help Keith learn braille so that he could read? "Why, I could read to him or we could get someone to record books on a tape recorder so that Keith could listen when he wanted to," he thought. The counselor had also said something about a "talking-book machine" and a library for blind people. Maybe Keith could attend his same school and be with his friends; they'd help him. But he'd get less out of so many activities like the ball games, and he had been looking forward so to track and had even talked about trying to play basketball now that he was in junior high. Those things would never be possible now, but maybe they could run—if he built a guidewire out in the backyard. Despite his loss of vision, Keith could still run, and maybe they could even figure out a way for him to run on the track at school. He'd talk to the coach about that. Life wasn't going to be exactly the same, but he and his wife could help Keith find other ways to pursue most of the same interests and responsibilities.

Then he remembered how quiet Keith had been recently; all he wanted to do was sit in his room and listen to music. He wondered if the boy's behavior was a reflection of his own sadness. He resolved to change his attitude, and perhaps Keith would gradually become the adventuresome boy he had been before the accident.

As he went upstairs to join his wife, Keith's father had a greater sense of peace. His mind was beginning to clear and he knew now that they could all keep on living. Of course, he realized their lives would be different and there would always be times when he'd feel terrible and Keith would feel defeated, but they could talk together and reason things out, and somehow they'd find a way to face the future together—a changed future, but a challenging one.

Summary

These word pictures of four children who are visually handicapped illustrate the range of feeling, learning, and functioning associated with different characteristics and conditions. Children may be born totally blind and never feel the need for vision; others may have very little vision which they must learn to use; some may have adequate but impaired vision and suddenly begin to lose it; and a few may experience traumatic loss due to accidents or disease before they are grown. One characteristic they all share is parents who have certain feelings and thoughts about themselves and their children that will influence, and in some cases determine, the child's attitudes and feeling about himself.

Medical people are often matter-of-fact about the condition of the eye and its functioning, and either unable or uninclined to make helpful suggestions to parents regarding how they can help their children. Except for the fact of being visually handicapped, the children may have few other qualities in common in relation to their social, emotional, mental, or personal development. Each child's potential for learning to function optimally within his family, school, or in the broader social environment may be fostered or inhibited by the attitudes of the people and the factors within those settings.

Carl's behavior, for example, was similar in many ways to that of any totally blind three-year-old who had learned to function with what resources he had and was oblivious to what he did not have. He had learned to use his other senses in his own way. Carl's mother had adjusted her interactions and relations to his patterns of learning. She had obviously included him in her activities in the home and had patiently explained things to him. It was evident also that she had managed him and corrected him as she would have any child. When he had wanted to help, she had let him; therefore, he had learned to recognize all household objects and the sounds associated with them. Although her expectations of him were never beyond what he was capable of doing, he had been included.

But their life hadn't always been so. At first Carl had cried frequently and had been very active. The parents had soon understood his need for more attention and tried to include him in their activities. Because of their encouragement and attentions he had been able to organize his world as he knew it and to achieve a feeling of comfort within it. As Carl gained greater control over his actions and some knowledge about what he wanted to do, he was able to find his own ways to solve problems. Frequent interpretation through verbal explanation was necessary to help him sort out his experiences and use this information to expand his repertoire of behavioral responses and to structure his knowledge about the world.

During his early development, Carl was dependent on others for interpretation and reinforcement, but by the time he entered school, he had acquired some control over his environment and was able to function with considerable independence. The attitudes he developed about himself and his relationships with others were determined largely by the attitudes of his parents toward him and their accepting him as he was. At first they were anguished, insecure, and sometimes sad—feelings that were normal under the circumstances. But determination, love for their child, and confidence in their ability to meet life's problems enabled them to learn the meaning of accepting realities that they could not change. They read everything available about blind children and adjusted their lives and interactions with Carl as his needs seemed to indicate. There would always need to be special ways for him to learn some things, and he would require a longer time and a greater effort to learn certain functional skills throughout his life.

In contrast, Lucy was thought of as a seeing child, since her parents hoped and looked for evidence of her ability to see. There were some commonalities between Carl and Lucy in that both were functioning in relation to the resources they had, never having known the sight they should or could have had. Her parents learned to make minor adjustments to assist Lucy in clarifying the distortions and confusions that arose constantly. The many contradictions in her behavior presented conflicting evidence about the nature of her vision, but such contradictions exist in the cases of many "low-vision" children, and few definitive predictions can be made about their potential for learning and development.

Those around Lucy came to be observant and perceptive of her efforts to use her vision and began to encourage her continually to look. For Lucy, this stimulated an attitude of searching for clarification of a distorted and bewildering world, in which she could learn to feel comfortable and secure. Nevertheless, her behavior indicated that she was a seeing child and could continue to develop greater visual efficiency as modifications were made for her and as she, in turn, made the adjustments compatible with her ability.

The flexibility and tremendous capacity for adjustment inherent in all children cannot be overemphasized. The discussion of Dora clearly illustrates these abilities to adjust. In Dora's case, the challenge was primarily for her parents and teachers to reinforce her positive attitudes and motivation, being careful not to interfere in the adjustment to losing her vision by stressing their concern or by imposing adult fears on the child. The possibility of making a gradual transition from performing as a seeing child to performing as a blind child meant that she would have more time to adjust to her visual loss and could use her remaining visual capabilities for support, as she began to develop new styles of learning. The fact that she could use remembered visual imagery to help her associate and integrate new learning patterns and skills, in addition to having been around other children who were totally blind and whom she accepted as her friends, made it easier for her to continue to consider herself a capable person who would be able to find ways to cope satisfactorily.

In contrast, the sudden and traumatic loss of vision in Keith's case, combined with the conditions of the accident, posed a somewhat different type of challenge for both Keith and his parents. Adjusting to his blindness could take longer and be a more tumultuous experience for him. Parental and peer attitudes would have a strong effect on the speed and quality of his accepting himself and his limitations, as his father began to realize. Parental guilt or sorrow would be significant influences in the adjustment process of a twelve-year-old boy. With the support and understanding of peers, parents, and teachers, Keith could continue to recall many visual memories and use them as a basis for adapting and modifying his life. Clearly, there would be some difficulties as he tried to adapt to totally different ways of learning, using new media and equipment. No doubt he would experience periods of frustration and even regression as he searched for different ways to accomplish what he formerly did with ease.

A new pattern of thinking and functioning would be required not only of Keith, but a reorganized way of life with many modifications and adaptations would also be necessary for the entire family. Naturally, future vocational and occupational interests and goals would have to be redirected and reevaluated. Because of emotional stress, demands on the boy's affective behavior would take precedence for a short time; as functional accommodations were made, then more time and energy would be available for reorganizing thinking and behavior in the reach toward adulthood.

Throughout the text, specific factors from each of the cases just described will be recalled and related to discussions, where appropriate. At times, the child (in referring to his or her impairment) may be identified by name. More frequently, the reader will be free to make his own associations and inferences.

2 Confusion in Words; Clarity in Concepts

Words are not reality, nor can they describe reality; but words can change our understanding of reality. Words used as labels or as terms to describe people may often have the effect of assigning people to a group to which they may or may not belong, thereby ignoring other individual characteristics that may differentiate an individual from all other members of the group. Labels or descriptive words used in referring to children may imply that there is something undesirable *within* the child, creating a difference greater than exists in reality.

Historical Terminology

As far back as the early 1800s, there has been a lack of precision in the use of terms relating to those who have visual impairments or who are totally without sight. The inconsistency in the use of terms by doctors, psychologists, and educators may be characteristic of professional or cultural attitudes, different concerns among the various disciplines, and also of the divergent roles to which each discipline is assigned. These divergent roles and attitudes reflect the confusion that has resulted from the lack of agreement in terminology, even among professionals directly associated daily with persons who are blind or have impaired vision. The list of terms that appears below illustrates that even within each discipline has existed a variety of labels, used over the last 150 years, for describing visual handicaps.

medically blind	visually handicapped
economically blind	partially seeing
braille blind	visually defective
educationally blind	visually disabled
functionally blind	visually impaired
congenitally blind	visually limited

adventitiously blind	low vision
legally blind	residual vision
partially blind	subnormal vision
vocationally blind	

Educational programs for those with visual problems and the words used to describe these programs have experienced similarly inconsistent labelling: sight-saving, vision or sight conservation, partially seeing, braille blind, and more recently, visually handicapped. Perhaps this multitude of words to talk about children with impaired vision has limited the planning of more appropriate educational programs; certainly the confusion in terminology has been a deterrent to gathering precise information through research. Many of the following questions are yet to be answered through consistent study and further information gathering.

1. How much vision is enough vision?
2. What constitutes a visual handicap in learning?
3. What are the critical variables influencing individual visual behavior in children?
4. Why is it that some children with severe visual impairments function at markedly higher levels than others who have much less severe impairments?
5. Is it the visual impairment itself or other impinging factors that limit the development, learning, and functioning in children?
6. What is the relation (if any) between impairment in the visual sense and what one can learn to see?

Current Terminology

During recent years, there appears to have been a movement among optometric and medical specialists and educators to refine the terminology and definitions to minimize possible confusion. For the purpose of identifying with greater clarity each individual's needs and specific behavioral characteristics, negative, misleading, and contradictory terms must be eliminated.

The term *visually handicapped* is being used widely at present to denote the total group of children who have impairments in the structure or functioning of the visual sense organ—the eye—irrespective of the nature and extent of the impairment. This term has gained acceptance because the impairment causes a limitation that, even with the best possible correction, interferes with incidental or normal learning through the sense of vision (Taylor, 1973, p. 156) and constitutes a handicap. Throughout the rest of this book, *visually handicapped* will be used to refer to the total group of children who require special educational provisions because of visual problems. Such a definition is quite appropriate for educational purposes and should be encouraged to differentiate children's learning and developmental needs from those of adults, who may have additional or entirely different legal, vocational, and medical factors to consider.

Since *visually handicapped* does not distinguish individual differences within this total group of children, more specific terms may be useful to the educator. Although the terms and definitions that follow may not be acceptable to all educators, they may help to provide some clarity and consistency in thinking about children and their specific learning needs. Only these terms will be used in the discussions throughout this text (except when quoted statements from others include different words).

Blind.   This term will be used to refer to children who have only light perception without projection, or those who are totally without the sense of vision (Faye, 1970). A child may be *blind at birth* (as in the case of Carl), or a child may lose vision sometime during his school years and *be blinded* either by an accident or by disease (as in the cases of Keith and Dora). Educationally, the blind child is one who learns through braille and related media without the use of vision (Halliday, 1970), although perception of light may be present and useful in orientation and movement.

Low vision.   Children who have limitations in distance vision but are able to see objects and materials when they are within a few inches or at a maximum of a few feet away are another subgroup. Most low-vision children will be able to use their vision for many school learning activities, a few for visual reading perhaps, whereas others may need to use tactual materials and possibly even braille to supplement printed and other visual materials. For some purposes and under varying conditions relative to light and personal characteristics, such children will always need to be made aware of what they are able to see and given assistance and encouragement in looking at educational materials and other objects (as in the case of Lucy). Under no circumstances should low-vision children be referred to as "blind."

Visually limited.   This term refers to children who in some way are limited in their use of vision under average circumstances. They may have difficulty seeing learning materials without special lighting, or they may be unable to see distant objects unless the objects are moving, or they may need to wear prescriptive lenses or use optical aids and special materials to function visually. Visually limited children will be considered for all educational purposes and under all circumstances as seeing children.

These terms shall be used to refer to the three major groupings within the broad range of visually handicapped children. The additional terms defined below will be useful to the reader in the discussions throughout the text. These terms will always be used in the manner defined.

Visual acuity.   "Acuity" refers to a clinical measurement of the ability to discriminate clearly the fine details of objects or symbols at a specified distance.

Visual impairment.   This term denotes any clinically diagnosable deviation in the structure or functioning of the tissues or parts of the eye. The impairment may be in the central part of the eye, such as the lens or the area around the macula, in which case the person could have very good peripheral vision but have trouble seeing fine detail. Conversely, the impairment might be in the structure or cells in the peripheral area, often causing what is referred to as "tunnel vision," and the person could have very clear central vision at a specific point of focus but could not see to either side.

Visual perception.   This term will be used to mean the ability to interpret what is seen, that is, the ability to understand and interpret meaningfully all information received through the visual sense. Information coming through the eyes must be received in the brain and coded and associated with other information. Even in cases of impairment or when acuity is poor, the brain receives visual impressions and is able to interpret them quite accurately.

> It is not the poor vision that causes poor learning, but it is what the brain does with the visual data. It must be intact in order to make sense of various stimuli, to store up experience, to see symbols and know what they mean, to remember and associate printed letters and words. The eye does not have to be intact, but the associative areas of the brain must be. (Faye, 1970, p. 137)

Visual perception is a decision process that is related more to the child's learning capabilities than to the condition of the eyes.

Visual functioning.   This term is used to denote how a person uses whatever vision he may have. Some children have very limited visual capability but use what vision they have so effectively that their functioning appears to be visually oriented. Others having similar visual potential are not aware of, or are not responsive to, visual stimuli and behave as if they were unable to see at all. Such children have probably been taught that they are blind, and therefore function accordingly. Visual functioning is related in part to the condition of the eye. More explicitly, visual functioning is determined by the experiences, motivations, needs, and expectations of each individual in relation to whatever visual capacity is available to satisfy curiosity and accomplish activities for personal satisfaction.

Visual efficiency.   This term is the most inclusive of all terms relating to vision and is contingent on many personal and environmental variables. Visual acuity at distance and at near, control of eye movements, accommodative and adaptive capabilities of the visual mechanism, speed and filtering abilities of the transmitting channels, and speed and quality of the processing ability of the brain are all related to visual efficiency. For educational purposes, visual efficiency is the most important consideration (Barraga, 1973). Visual efficiency is unique to each child and cannot be measured or predicted clinically with any accuracy by medical, psychological, or educational personnel.

Summary

To label as "blind" a child who is able to see many things is to imply that he is not expected to see, and in a short time he will begin to function as blind and perceive himself as incapable visually. Such ambiguous descriptions as "partially seeing" or "partially blind" seem to suggest a relationship between quantity of an attribute and quality of functioning in the individual—which is a false inference. However, to disregard all descriptive words would be foolish and possibly detrimental to children's safety as well as to their special learning needs. The words that are used should relate to development and learning in children.

From the long list of terms given at the beginning of this section, you will note that only those that have educational significance have been selected for use. The following educational definition is presented in a further attempt to encourage educators to "say what they mean and mean what they say":

> A visually handicapped child is one whose visual impairment interferes with his optimal learning and achievement, unless adaptations are made in the methods of presenting learning experiences, the nature of the materials used, and/or in the learning environment.

3

Early Encounters and Interactions

To accept any single theory of child development as the basis for discussing the early encounters and interactions of visually handicapped children would limit our perspective. Regardless of their primary focus, most developmentalists are concerned with the emotional-social, physical, and mental aspects of development and learning in children. The terms *affective, psychomotor,* and *cognitive* are being used widely to discuss these dimensions of development and learning. The discussions in the next four chapters will use these terms with the following meanings:

Affective: Feelings and attitudes about oneself and in relation to other people.
Psychomotor: The physical movement and control of the body in actions and interactions with the environment and in performance of skills.
Cognitive: The development of thought processes from the memory of actions and words to the use of symbolic language to express abstract ideas.

The central theme of this chapter on the visually handicapped child's early interactions is his affective development as it relates to, and to some extent establishes, the bases for his psychomotor and cognitive development. Many of the ideas for the thoughts to be discussed here have emerged from the research of Erikson (1972), Hunt (1961), Montessori (1967), Murphy (1972), and Piaget (1966, 1970, 1973).

When used to refer to children, the words *development* and *learning* may be considered synonymous. The emergence of the human being encompasses physiological maturation as well as learned behavior, and since much learning is dependent on a variety of developmental factors, to make a distinction between these two terms could introduce an artificial dichotomy. To avoid an implied bias toward either a hereditarian or an environmental point of view, *learning* and *development* will be used as mutually inclusive terms.

General Concepts of Affective Development

A generally accepted notion is that the process of development and learning in all children begins at birth and is related to their needs, feelings, and potential. Halliday (1970, p. 15) expresses the special significance of this idea for visually handicapped children in relation to their developmental needs:

> To be loved and to return love; to be able to trust both people and things which have meaning to them; to develop increasing trust in themselves; to be cared for and to care. . . . They must learn in all kinds of ways: through their senses, through play, through work, through exploration, through trial and error, and through being taught.

Because visually handicapped children are basically like all children, many of their needs are the same, despite the fact that the process and the nature of satisfying these needs for development and learning may require from parents some special knowledge and consistent attention.

The critical variables in interpersonal interactions and environmental encounters as foundations for development and learning focus on what happens to the child within his family. The child's affective development is largely contingent on the family's attitudes toward him and their personal involvement with him in his striving to become a human being.

> With his first breath at the moment of birth, an infant has the capacity to become a receiving, participating, interacting human being who enjoys a reciprocally satisfying relationship with his immediate environment, and eventually a fulfilling involvement with an ever-expanding world. (Barraga, 1973, p. 117)

Parental nurturance.   In the first few days of life, every touch, every word, every person, and every object encountered may have affective meaning to the infant. If we accept the idea that all infants experience internal stress from hunger and other physical discomforts, then the early reflexive movements appear to be generated from within the infant's own body. However, these reflexive movements quickly become integrated with responses generated by external stimulation from other people. Knight (1972) has suggested that perhaps the general purpose of all movement and behavior in infancy is to reduce tension. The primary role of the parents, then, is to create a feeling of peace, comfort, and confidence, which is achieved more readily through one significant person, usually the mother, as she touches, pats, strokes, and manipulates the infant. Not only does this continual cuddling provide a basis for establishing trust and security, but it may also supply the framework from which the infant organizes these sensations into a "cognitive map of himself"

(Murphy, 1972), that is, knowing that he exists within a larger environment. The reciprocal exchanges in touch give the infant feelings of enjoyment from receiving attention and, in addition, the mutual activity between adult and infant creates a desire in the infant to explore and discover. When given the opportunity to do so, the infant quickly begins to gain some control over his own movement responses.

The infant's responses to nurturance and play have a strong influence on the quality and nature of the interaction. Blind babies cannot see facial expressions or other positive indications of adult satisfactions and are less likely to interact in ways that are motivating to parents. Passivity or lack of expected responses could lead adults to think that the baby was not enjoying the cuddling and play. Parents must learn to look for other indicators of pleasure in the blind infant and search for different ways to generate responses other than those related to visual interactions. More touching and handling of the baby is necessary to help the infant *feel* the interaction rather than see it.

If he fails to develop strong affectional ties and pleasure in human contacts, the blind baby will remain at a primitive level of affective development, constantly seeking and exploiting any source of comfort available to him. Body play, or manipulation, helps the infant learn new patterns of body movement and minimizes the need for stereotyped and rigid tension-reducing movements—for example, such bizarre motions as aimless waving of arms, rocking the body back and forth, poking the fists into the eyes, or shaking the head—which become resistant to change after several months. Emotional security and lessened anxiety seem to reduce the need for these movements and the frequency of their occurrence. The frequent labelling of such behaviors as "blindisms" is erroneous, since the same actions may be observed in sighted babies who are deprived of emotional needs and adequate nurturance.

If a baby begins to feel that he cannot influence his own world or effect some control over what happens to him, he is likely to begin to retreat from the world and those within it. A certain cognitive satisfaction relates to the development of a strong self involved in "making things happen" and in mastering the environment, to say nothing of the mediating effect that this satisfaction may have on later cognitive development. Piaget (1966, 1973) suggests that feelings begin to supply the energy necessary for action and for specifying goals for behavior; these "feeling-oriented" actions may be related to the development of conscious thought. In time, the infant, the baby, and eventually the young child learns that he is somebody who can *do* many things. Eventually he feels that he can function in his own way, "at his *own* pace, exploring his *own* interests, for his *own* purposes" (Weber, 1971). Having achieved this level of affective development, the child is well on the way to knowing who he is, what he is about, and to use feelings, actions, and thoughts to direct future learning.

Affective Development in the Visually Handicapped Child

With these general concepts of child development in mind, let us now turn our attention to the visually handicapped child, who because of his impairment may have less opportunity to experience the emergence of a strong identity of self and understanding of feelings. Just as Carl's and Lucy's parents probably were upset, parents are naturally distressed when they learn that they have a blind baby or a baby who has a serious visual impairment. Most parents experience similar feelings, although they may feel guilty about acknowledging them even to themselves or to each other. Because of the anxiety and insecurity in not knowing how to accept this unexpected (and unasked for) "different" baby, they may be overwhelmed by the diagnosis of the impairment and forget, momentarily at least, that this is a real, live baby who needs them and their love in the same way that a "normal" baby would. Not knowing exactly what to do or being afraid of doing the wrong thing, parents may have a tendency to leave the baby alone except to provide physical care, while they try to struggle with their own feelings. Being left alone defeats the need of the visually handicapped child to achieve the first level of affective development—human attachment.

Body manipulation.   With the visually handicapped infant, body play must replace eye play to communicate maternal concern and love—the facilitators of developing a self-concept. More than the usual amount of time should be spent cuddling, holding, touching, stroking, and moving the baby. At the same time, soothing, comforting sounds and words from the parents will help establish love bonds through a "tactile, auditory language" (Fraiberg, Smith, and Adelson, 1969) instead of the usual attachment established through eye contact. Human interactions provide the basis for the infant's future learning; therefore, a dialogue of signals and responses between the baby and the parents is essential. If the visually handicapped child does not experience this interaction, his personal security in relating to others and eventually to his world is reduced.

Sound stimulation.   Parents of the visually handicapped infant may have to find new ways of expressing their own feelings of pleasure when interacting with their child. In a few short months, as parents satisfy this hunger for cuddling, holding, touching, and moving, the baby will begin to respond and show feelings of pleasure and comfort. In addition, the infant learns to make an association between the human voice and the tactual intimacy. Once this association has been made, the human voice from a distance and without physical touching begins to unite the child with his world, forming a basis for experiencing feelings from voice and environmental sounds alone. Parents can continue to talk about every sound that is heard and every movement that is made so that sounds and actions begin to have meanings to the blind child comparable to those acquired incidentally through vision for the child who can see.

Developing affective relationships.   With strong human attachments to comfort and strengthen him, the visually handicapped child is better equipped to cope with the world of mysterious objects that he often encounters accidentally and that seem to come "out of nowhere and disappear into nothingness" once he has lost contact with them (Fraiberg et al., 1969). Sustained by a feeling of security and encouraged by concerned others, the world becomes a friendly rather than a fearful place, and the toddler is ready to explore, to learn to control, and to act on the world beyond his own body.

We must remember that feelings and desires are closely related to movement and action; and because sound and tactile sensations do not have the same arousing and motivating effects as do visual sensations, without consistent interaction and stimulation, the visually handicapped child may become passive. The inactivity, occasioned by no one to talk with him and nothing meaningful to touch, creates the need for the undesirable repetitive and stereotyped movements referred to earlier. Interestingly, none of these stereotyped behaviors is noticed in blind children in Africa, where mothers carry their infants on their backs all day, talk to them, and include them constantly as part of the complete world of the family. You may recall that none of these behaviors was observed in Carl, who was apparently emotionally secure and trusted himself and others.

Recent research in ego disturbances suggests that these disruptive patterns of affective development probably have their beginnings during the first eighteen months of life. The visually handicapped infant or toddler may have feelings of rejection or of living in a world void of stimuli if he is left by himself for prolonged periods with no tactual or auditory contacts, even though there may be warm and accepting feelings in those around him. The immobile baby who has vision can satisfy this need for sensory input by looking at things, learning to focus his eyes, trying to reach out and touch; during these periods he is learning eye-hand coordination. Not equipped with this ability, the visually handicapped child relies on sustained sound contacts to keep him in touch with the world.

During the first eighteen months, toys should have a strong tactual appeal, with a variety of pleasant textures. Later, when the baby is more active, toys capable of making sounds may be added to encourage the child to follow the sound with his hand. This ear-hand coordination in effect becomes a substitute for the eye-hand coordination of the baby who sees, but more importantly, ear-hand coordination becomes critical in later months, when sound localization and spatial orientation are important for purposeful movement. Carl, at four, used sound and spatial cues very effectively as he located his toys and moved about the house and even outside. Remember, though, that he also sought verbal or tactual reassurance frequently to feel continued security and to maintain contact with others.

Parents and siblings form the basic psychosocial (social-emotional) climate for the development of positive affective behavior through emotional interaction. A close relationship with loving others enables the child to satisfy his needs, after which he is able to gain a sense of inner control and begin to cope with his own feelings, in addition to responding to feelings elicited by loving others. The picture of Carl revealed a child who had the opportunity for strong social and emotional interactions in his first years, which prepared him to progress to the psychomotor phase of development.

However, it would be misleading to suggest that Carl's affective development was complete or would ever be fully realized. Psychosocial development must be fostered and expanded throughout life in order to maintain one's mental health. Although stresses and frustrations are a natural part of life for everyone, for the visually handicapped child, the alternatives available for coping with stresses and for reducing tension and anxiety may be restricted by environmental conditions and societal attitudes and expectations. Consequently, chances for developing and maintaining a flexible, adaptable concept of self are strengthened when the child's early years in the family and in school have provided stable patterns of interaction.

The effects of deprivation.   The discussion presented thus far has revolved almost exclusively around the positive aspects of affective development, focusing on the critical early years of social interaction. Let us compare positive development with some of the possible effects of depriving the severely visually handicapped child of adequate social and emotional interactions. To begin with, the lack of verbal interaction may have a retarding effect on all dimensions of development, but more especially on that of social communication through speech and language. Passively exposing a severely visually handicapped child to an auditory environment such as family conversation, household noises, radio, or television without personalized interpretation could have negative consequences. Echolalic, or repetitive, speech frequently develops in children who are blind. This imitative speech may take the form of repetition of jingles or commercial tunes. But the imitation of sounds or simply saying words without understanding them does not indicate language acquisition, nor does such behavior foster sequential development in higher cognitive levels.

The sounds and words heard and repeated from passive exposure never become important as a means of social communication with another person. Interpersonal communication through language is one of the strong forces in the socialization process, because feelings are both expressed and received more vividly through verbal interaction. For the child who cannot see facial expressions, gestures, and the other subtleties conveyed through body language, the feelings communicated through voice are most meaningful.

Visually handicapped children may develop bizarre behavioral patterns as a means of getting attention and satisfying their unmet affective needs. In fact, some children are able to manipulate adults so adroitly that they exercise almost complete control over their environments, although the attention they receive is not the kind that helps them develop socially. Could it be that these children feel themselves puppets maneuvered through life without understanding how or why?

Summary

Failure to recognize the potency of language interaction in the personal and social development of visually handicapped children may have lasting inhibitory consequences on the psychosocial aspects of personality throughout school and adult life. When a child shares his feelings and thoughts verbally with an adult, and that adult responds in a similar manner, the child realizes that his thoughts and feelings are accepted by others and are significant to them. This does not mean that the adult bombards the child verbally, talking about things without appropriate tactual contact, but rather that the adult listens as the child talks about his own impressions and talks only to verify or to correct inaccuracies in the child's perceptions. Experiencing and sharing in frequent verbal interactions helps the child know that he is a person who can acquire information for himself, and that he has worth and value to another.

Satisfaction in human relationships frees the child to recognize that he possesses a self independent of others. He can be autonomous and search actively to encounter and relate to the world of concrete objects. Movement and activity bring the child into contact with things over which he begins to exercise control, which thrusts him into the dimension of psychomotor behavior—the topic for the next chapter.

4

Movement, Exploration, and Spatial Awareness

The previous chapter focused on the importance of creating feelings of security and trust in the infant and young child through human interaction. A sense of security provides a stable basis for the desire and motivation to "reach out" and extend the self into the world of objects. Chapter 3 suggested also that the rhythmic involuntary movements seem to be related to the infant's internal affective feelings as well as to relieving tension originating within the infant. These reactions to tension through movement are considered responses to the "biological impetus" within the infant and not solely responses to outside stimulation; as such, they may enable the organism to record motor patterns at a very early age (Furth, 1969; Hebb, 1949).

Early Movement

Movement at this stage permits the infant to contact the environment with his body, although unintentionally at first. Later he becomes aware of the object world as a basis for self-initiated, goal-directed movement. These early movements begin to have meaning when the infant accepts them into his own body and uses them to structure and control future movements. In translating Piaget's ideas, Furth (1969) says that this internalization is one of the first stages of "knowing" or learning. He suggests further that any functional exchange between the moving infant and the environment provides the sensorimotor integration that is essential for perceptual development, since movement helps the child define, integrate, and understand his body as it interacts with the environment so that he becomes a feeling, moving, and thinking being. This most elemental perceptual knowledge is the result of a mental organizing activity interacting with sensory information, since "a thing in the world is not an object of knowledge until the knowing organism interacts with it and constitutes it as an object" (Furth, 1969, p. 19).

After patterns of movement have begun to be established, and the infant knows because of his previous actions that things exist outside of himself and apart from him, motor activities may become goal oriented—that is, there is a purpose in movement such as to make contact with a person or object or to change body position or the position of a single body part. Hence, these primitive psychomotor actions form the groundwork for the later coordinated movements of manipulation, locomotion, and skill development.

Movement and vision.   When vision is present, it is the first sense to make contact with the environment beyond the body itself. From the time the sighted infant begins to hold his eyes open, light is all around him, and the stimulation of the visual sense from this point on is virtually constant. As early as the first few weeks of life, infants have been observed to attempt to focus on, and respond to, patterns and colors. Visual stimulation is thought to excite the organism, and indeed, babies engage in very active movement behavior when looking at stimulating visual patterns.

The extent to which vision is actually a stimulating and facilitating factor in affective, psychomotor, perceptual, and cognitive development is not known precisely. Whether vision promotes movement or whether movement promotes visual search and control is not yet determined; however, there are many indications that sensorimotor development proceeds with greater rapidity when the reciprocal action between vision and movement is optimal. Clearly, movement toward an object is more likely to occur when the object can be seen, and certainly the child's movement through space is more likely to occur when he sees something of interest toward which he wishes to move.

Vision, even without movement, offers opportunities for looking at the world and provides a wide variety of vicarious experiences that become part of the child's knowledge of the world. Vision not only extends the quantity of information available but also provides unique sensory data that are never quite as accurate when gathered through another sense. Specific details of form, color, and the spatial relationships between objects can be perceived only through vision. In addition, vision provides an instant concept of totality of what one sees and is thought by many to be the prime unifier of all the other sensory information acquired during the early months and years. Visual images held in the brain provide a constant referent system for recall, even after the objects are no longer visible. An impression of the constancy of the world and of the objects in it is achieved readily through the visual sense but remains variable when perceived through other senses only. Vision permits the child early learning through imitation in actions and the ability to refine the coordination of his body with what he sees.

Movement with impaired vision.   If there is a strong interrelationship between movement and learning, then for children who are blind or have low vision, movement may be the most accurate replacement for vision in clarifying information about the world. Perhaps physical movement alone, if carefully designed, could facilitate the same quality of psychomotor development as that achieved by children who have both vision and movement.

For all visually handicapped children, external visual stimulation for spontaneous movement, exploration, and spatial awareness will be greatly diminished or totally lacking from birth. The manner in which visually handicapped children organize perceptions and learn through other senses will be different from that of a child who has vision and will depend on those around the child to teach movement and to provide the desire and reason for exploration. Since the needs and problems of the totally blind child differ somewhat from those of the low-vision child, we will first discuss the totally blind child, using Carl (described in Chapter 1) as an example. The aspects of psychomotor development unique to the low-vision child will refer back to the picture of Lucy, also presented in the first chapter.

Psychomotor Development in Blind Children

Van Weelden (1967) says that the body in action defines space and organizes it into a perception of personal space. Others have suggested that space exists for blind persons only to the extent that the body or some part of it has moved through space. This movement involves the muscular system, and through its use a kinesthetic awareness, or a "feel," is perceived and internalized. Knowledge of this nature may be referred to as "muscle sense." The responsibility for parents, who are the first educators, and eventually for teachers, is to foster as much as possible this internalization of kinesthetic information—by moving the baby's arms and legs in up, down, and circular motions to imitate reaching, turning, and stepping—for use in later exploration and independent movement.

Body image.   The work of Cratty (1971) emphasizes the need for developing "body image" in blind children, because the body for the blind child is the "center platform" from which all knowledge of movement and space is acquired. The blind person must know about his own body, how it can move, his potential for exerting control over movement, and his body's relationship to other objects and persons in space.

In the blind infant, the first awareness of body parts comes through movement of the extremities (hands and feet) to touch another part. Movement from one body section to another promotes the development of "motor patterns." If this structured manipulation is not done for the infant, primitive motor behaviors will persist into childhood as purposeless mannerisms, a subject discussed in the previous chapter.

Using the hands to find head, feet, shoulders, and other body parts stabilizes the infant's orientation in "near space," which is critical to freedom of body movement through "extended space." The hands become finely developed instruments of investigation essential for tactual exploration and the manipulation skills required in later learning. The feel of motion helps to replace the inability to see motion. The parents' constant use of words to identify the part of the body being touched is necessary to develop an awareness in the child that there are names for different body areas, in addition to establishing a kinesthetic image of the body as a related and constant whole capable of being regulated at will.

The tactual-kinesthetic awareness and stabilization of the object world is the next hurdle in the blind child's psychomotor development. The parents should make available every small and large object that is safe to touch or to explore and manipulate, as the child begins to show interest in both inanimate and living things. Removing objects from the blind child's surroundings for the sake of protecting the objects from falling or breaking creates a sterile environment from which he can gather no information. Confining a child who can't see to a crib or playpen after he has begun to crawl or toddle about is a further obstacle to his learning. Encouragement and freedom to explore and move about are indispensable for providing a range and variety of experiences necessary for all facets of development and also for future success in academic endeavors.

Permitting the blind child to encounter the same bumps, bruises, falls, and other natural consequences of independent actions that all children experience is difficult for some parents. The common inclination is to protect such a "helpless" child from a seemingly hostile world, but to do so communicates to him feelings of inadequacy and incompetence and makes him needlessly dependent.

Two important skills can be developed through freedom to move about the house: the use of the total body as it moves through space to encounter stationary (and usually larger) objects, and the use of the hands to explore objects that are either stable or that move with contact. The parents' attaching words to describe the body action and the objects will help the child interpret the nature of things and the body function required to control his movements among them.

Without vision to cause him to imitate the body movements of others, the blind child must experience the movement in his own muscles before he can know that a specific action is possible or understand verbal instructions from others. Hearing actions described has no meaning to the young blind child unless he is simultaneously performing the action with his own body.

Many of the postural deviations and infantile patterns of movement observed in numerous blind children could be prevented by the use of simple instructions, such as "head up," "shoulders back," "long steps, " and "swinging arms." There are specific exercises designed to accentuate body image and movement to promote overall coordination of the body in stationary positions as well as in locomotion. For example, *Movement without Sight* (Kratz, 1973) contains a variety of suggestions for physical activities, dances, and games for visually handicapped children.

Thinking back to Carl and how easily and with specific purpose he was able to move around the house and outside, one may infer that his parents taught him about his body and its use from early infancy. They may have done this by moving his body in all possible ways, turning it in every position, moving individual limbs and parts through space to develop his kinesthetic sense, and by stroking and touching his body with different textures to stimulate his awareness of the multitude of possible sensations and perceptions. Carl's parents worked to teach him to hold his head in an upright position in order to gain muscular control of the head and neck, since the blind child has no reason to hold his head in an upright position in order to see. In addition, his parents probably played many hand and finger and other body-part games with him, which enabled him to learn to position his body in relation to theirs.

By the time Carl was four or five months old, his parents were probably propping him in a sitting position and playing with him on their laps to promote the strengthening of head, neck, and trunk muscles, as well as helping him expand his world by hearing sounds from different distances and locations and by learning to manipulate objects with his own body. When he was able to sit alone, by six or eight months of age, he was probably given a "controlled space" (Fraiberg and Adelson, 1973) in which he could find many interesting objects. According to Fraiberg and Adelson, blind babies exhibited exploration and recognition qualities through handling and manipulating the object world as early as eight months. From observing Carl, it seems apparent that he was given much guidance and frequent demonstration of how to use objects, in addition to explanations of the effects of his actions on them. For blind children, nursery rhymes that use body manipulation substitute for picture books. Again, if he had not been encouraged to search and find objects or given adequate body manipulation, he might have become inactive and passive and sought stimulation through his own body, which would have caused him to exhibit the meaningless movements described earlier.

The objects offered the child for play at this period in development should be simple in form and shape, varied in textures and weight, and capable of some auditory feedback to encourage the child to develop ear-hand-brain coordination as a substitute for the eye-hand coordination developed by normally seeing children. Toys and objects that change their form when pushed or pressed on, so long as the child is encouraged to use hand and finger movements to lift and press and move such objects, provide perceptions that are necessary for more refined tactual discrimination and recognition, which will be discussed later in this chapter. Such structured play gave Carl the knowledge necessary to organize and reorganize mentally the objects in relation to himself and his ability to act on them, and also taught him a reality and a constancy similar to that acquired by children who are able to see.

Having gained some control of his body, a perception of space from movement through it, and a perception of objects in relation to himself, Carl developed at a normal age the muscular coordination and strength to hold his body in an upright position (for the most part) and to walk and move in purposeful directions. As he began to move, he was probably able to perceive through the echoes bouncing off walls and off near and far objects the position of his body in relation to those objects, enabling him to avoid them as he moved. At first, of course, Carl was given much guidance, encouragement, and physical contact. His parents may even have stood him on their own feet and walked with him for him to get the feel of movement of his body through space. Familiar toys that made a sound were probably used to get him to move toward them to touch and manipulate them. Because of previous experiences in having his body moved and in learning to move it himself, his kinesthetic memory developed, giving him the ability to determine his position and to use selected external cues from the things he encountered, permitting him to begin to move on his own.

Spatial orientation.   With practice, the blind child learns "to assimilate these signals into a meaningful conceptual model of space" (Kidwell and Greer, 1973, p. xvi). Lydon and McGraw (1973) suggest that four aspects of spatial concepts form the basis for concept development in blind children: (1) action space with the body as a fixed point from which to anchor movements, (2) body space in which short distances can be measured in relation to body movement, (3) object space as the area within which awareness and location of objects can be perceived without actual contact, and (4) map space which is the mental organization of certain spatial areas in relation to the body.

Piaget would probably say that Carl had a cognitive map of himself and his surrounding world and was beginning to develop a style of learning that was unique for him. If he had lacked the opportunity to form these perceptions from birth and throughout the early learning years, Carl would most likely not have acquired the freedom of movement and purposeful manipulative skills evident from his behavior. He had learned to move efficiently without vision.

When a blind child enters a school learning situation lacking the early developmental skills more easily acquired before five or six years of age, the retarding effects are likely to be long lasting and possibly permanent. In such a case, achieving ease and efficiency in independent travel may never be possible, and the negative influence on developing abstract cognitive skills may be noticeable throughout life.

Assuming that Carl had taken walks with his parents and accompanied them on shopping tours, he would have developed numerous perceptions of the vast world of space and the information available for use in later learning. If his parents described to him such landmarks as lamp posts, mail boxes, buildings, curbs, and gutters, then he would be able to understand and follow instructions for independent mobility at school and in adult life.

Talking about the differences in textures of grass, gravel, cement, or sand while walking through them would develop a vocabulary necessary to progress in academic subjects. Unless such words as *inclines, slants, hills,* and *valleys* are "felt" through body awareness, they have no meaning to blind children. Expanding knowledge through using the body, combined with verbal interpretation, is the key to continuous refinement in motor skills for blind children and youth throughout their lives. Many affective problems could be avoided through greater focus on "action with words."

Reliance on Low Vision or Visual Imagery for Movement

Warren (1974, p. 161) postulates that, "Having vision simultaneously with the motor function allows registration of the motor function and its effects in a visual framework." Recalling the description of Lucy in comparison to the discussion of Carl, one can easily see that there are obvious differences in the psychomotor development of a child who has even limited visual capacity. Despite the discrepancies in her behavior in relation to her use of vision and the confusions in her movement patterns, the fact that she moved her body in relation to light and that she attempted to reach out away from her body when she was visually aware that objects were present indicate that she was using what little vision was available to her to guide movement. Her spontaneous awareness of visual space was, and would continue to be, limited to a very small area surrounding her body, but the fact that she was able to see objects and movement within this space permitted her to develop an awareness that there was something beyond her body.

As her parents encouraged her and enticed her to continue to move and explore, the more accurate she became in her movements and the greater curiosity she had about the blurred world she saw—but toward which she could move to gain a clearer impression. Crawling or toddling toward a wall mirror may have contributed to body awareness and body image. In this movement, she learned to gauge distance, even though she could not actually acquire a clear visual picture of what was in the distance. Although she knocked over objects, bumped into, and stumbled over things she could not see clearly, she was learning to correct herself. This behavior forged motor patterns into her nervous system, which would be key factors in her developing greater and greater independence in movement.

Of course, Lucy's parents were concerned and exercised some cautions, with good reason. Because of her lack of distance vision and the blurred nature of the environment she was experiencing, Lucy's safety was an important consideration. Perhaps her parents suggested that she listen in order to help her clarify what she could not see, and that she learn to anticipate possible dangers so that her movements would be cautious without being fearful. Her orientation in, and relationship with, the environment was a more easily acquired ability for Lucy than for Carl. Her limited vision permitted her to stabilize her concepts of both near and extended space into integrated visual and motor patterns. Games such as rolling, bouncing, or hitting balls; crawling and walking up and down flights of stairs with and without assistance; and others requiring her to use her vision for accuracy in spatial position or prediction of spatial distances may have fostered her visual-motor organization.

Selecting playthings for nursery-age children with low vision is a matter for careful consideration. Attention to texture and shape is as important as for the blind child, but the color and light-reflecting qualities are equally important; in fact, toys that have highly visible differences are often preferred over those that make a noise.

Studies of children, youth, and adults blinded at different ages suggest that a relationship exists between the length of time vision was present in early life and the subsequent ability to perform increasingly complex tasks requiring spatial awareness and manipulative skill (Valvo, 1971; Warren, 1974). Personal observations indicate a noticeable difference in movement patterns between congenitally blind children and those who had vision for as limited a period as eighteen months to two years, which lends validity to Piaget's idea of an internalized sensorimotor integration through early movement experiences.

Since Dora had limited but adequate vision and Keith had normal vision during their developmental years, it is reasonable to assume that their movement and exploratory patterns were well developed before they lost their vision. Both had good visual imagery of space, understood the relationship of their body within space, had seen their bodies in various positions and knew what they could do, and had developed stable motor patterns and skills. In both their cases, the primary concern would be for them to adapt to the use of other senses to alert themselves about the world and to guide them in their movements, as they recalled their visual perception of spatial relations.

Provided that parents and teachers encourage them to continue independent movement, their self-confidence should return with some ease. However, if they should develop anxiety and fear because of restriction and overprotection imposed on them, their adaptation to the use of other senses would be much slower, and indeed the motivation for adaptation might be lost. Calling on previously established visual imagery and associating this imagery with new patterns of tactual and auditory information, things soon begin to feel like they looked or sounded, and a modified picture of the world would soon emerge.

Because Dora and Keith already knew the names of the parts of their bodies and also had the language associated with body position within their repertoire, they were especially attuned to following verbal instructions in relation to their new exploration and movement and could interpret and associate easily the descriptive language of others in relation to their remembered visual imagery. Continuing recall of visual imagery in the case of those who have become blinded is crucial. The more visual recall required of the person, the longer and more vivid the visual images will remain. Just like any other facet of thought, memories that are unused will soon lose their clarity. During the adaptive period, it is especially important that verbal instructions be used to assist Dora and Keith in their movements and that parents, peers, and teachers refrain from moving or physically guiding them. Independence and self-confidence are much more easily acquired if blinded children are assumed to be able to follow instructions and permitted to move independently, according to instructions. Applying the notion that success promotes success, the more these youths move and travel independently, the more rapidly confidence and efficiency will become a reality.

Differential Program Planning

Congenitally blind children whose early experiences have been similar to Carl's can enter into physical education activities with sighted children with minimal assistance and encouragement when given the opportunity to participate. As soon as they learn stationary landmarks and are shown the routes to follow, congenitally blind children will learn to travel alone within the classroom, around the building, and on the playground with efficiency and confidence. Given the assistance of a mobility instructor, they will be ready to begin some independent travel within the neighborhood and to and from school, on foot or by public transportation, by the time they complete elementary school. With travel instruction in high school, blind children with good motor development have the potential for efficient independent travel in unfamiliar areas in adult life.

However, not all blind children enter school with established patterns of motor development. Those who have been restricted either because of parental fear that they will hurt themselves or simply lack of knowledge about how to raise a blind child may know little about their own bodies and even less about the realities of the environment. Such underdeveloped blind children may require as long as two or more years of physical therapy, intensive exercise, daily excursions in the out-of-doors, and regular field trips, in addition to a concentrated program of concrete learning experiences in language and developmental concepts (Hapeman, 1967; Hill, 1970). Many children progress rapidly and are able to grasp formal abstract concepts as readily as those whose early development was less delayed. Others may have multiple disabilities in addition to blindness, which may limit learning potential (a topic discussed in the next chapter).

Unlike Lucy, some children with low vision may enter school having no awareness of their visual potential and behave as if they were unable to see anything. Their parents, having been told the child was blind (using medical-legal criteria), have made no effort to stimulate the child visually or to encourage the use of residual vision. For these low-vision children, a program similar to that proposed for underdeveloped blind children, with special emphasis on visual development, would be advantageous. In every experience and activity, the child would be encouraged to "look" so as to learn to coordinate his visual and motor systems and to begin to bring increased clarity and order to a world that has been confusing. Although not all low-vision children will become primarily "visual learners," increased visual efficiency will enhance movement patterns, motor coordination, and conceptual development (Barraga, 1964).

Because Dora and Keith both had vision in their preschool and early school years, their movement patterns developed normally as a matter of course. Not only will they retain a mental picture of the world of objects and space, but they will also unconsciously use the movement patterns internalized within their bodies, even when they no longer have sight. The primary focus in teaching these children will not be their learning *how* to move but instead will concentrate attention on the feel of movement and visual recall of spatial concepts, while they adapt to using ear-brain coordination (rather than the eyes) to orient themselves within space and to guide and direct movement.

Summary

There are obvious differences in freedom of movement, mobility within limited environments, and future independent travel among the congenitally totally blind, those with limited vision, and those who are blinded after having acquired these skills. These differences must be considered in relation to the learning process and the teaching technique, for which appropriate adaptations must be made. Spatial orientation and concept formation require a long and tedious learning process for the totally congenitally blind child. He will learn to use his other senses, but must be constantly encouraged and supported by adults, who carefully plan sequential experiences as he gradually acquires skills. The concepts he acquires will necessarily be different from those acquired through the use of vision. The potential for independent travel at a later age is directly proportional to the early learning experiences provided him by his parents, and to the extent to which they encourage him to reach out and be independent and knowledgeable in movement.

The child with very limited vision will be able to use that vision to enhance his knowledge of the world and his exploration patterns. Independence in movement will come more easily and with greater efficiency as he continues to develop. As with the congenitally blind child, independence in travel is closely related to the appropriate learning experiences and encouragement provided in the early years.

Children who lose vision after having established their concepts of the world and their movement patterns must learn to adapt these patterns through using other senses. The adaptation process may be slow in the beginning and is related to psychological factors within the children and in those around them. Independence in travel can be maintained through appropriate teaching procedures directed toward encouraging the acquisition of different skills for movement and travel. Mobility training programs must be adapted to each individual and designed specifically in relation to previous development and learning.

5

Multi-Impairments
in Body Systems

Visually handicapped children who have impairments in other body systems are not a new subject, but in the past few years, so-called multihandicapped children have received greater attention. Evidence from surveys and studies has indicated that a large percentage of visually handicapped children may have other medical or psychological conditions (Graham, 1968; Gruber and Moor, 1963; Lowenfeld, 1969; Wolf, 1967). The functional or developmental problems we have discussed in previous chapters were attributed to sensory deprivation or limited interaction with the environment.

In this chapter, we will direct our attention to children who have clinical or medically diagnosed impairments in some body system other than the visual system.

Before the current decade, any child who was severely visually handicapped and also had damage to other body systems at birth was likely to have been ignored by educators because of the "hopelessness" of medical intervention, or may have been institutionalized on the recommendation of a medical person shortly after birth, or may simply have been kept at home, given total care, and considered incapable of learning. In the 1970s, a general change in attitudes about handicapped persons, more concerned and knowledgeable medical personnel, the growth of preschool programs, and groups of intelligent, interested parents make the likelihood of any of these previous patterns' recurring less likely. The rubella (German measles) epidemic of 1963–64, which resulted in a population of several thousand deaf-blind children, many of whom have additional impairments, may have provided the strongest impetus for doing something about children who have serious problems.

Typical Multi-Impairments—
Three Primary Groups

There are three major types of multi-impairments that require discussion in relation to their effect on the various dimensions of development. They are all impairments beyond visual impairment that interfere with learning and developmental processes. The more typical multi-impairments can be illustrated through short descriptions.

1. Cerebral palsy-visually handicapped.   Betty was a premature baby presented in breech position and was unable to breathe readily or normally. Whether or not she would live was in doubt for several hours, even after oxygen was administered in large doses. That she had survived was reason for great rejoicing by the doctors and her parents. The consequences of her complicated birth were not evident until some time later.

2. Severe brain damage.   Paul was born to very young parents, neither of whom was robustly healthy. The entire pregnancy was difficult, and the mother suffered a number of illnesses that required large doses of several drugs both to prevent losing the baby and to improve her own poor health. The mother was quite small, and at the time of delivery, Paul was a very large baby. Labor was prolonged, and instruments were necessary to accomplish the birth. Although the baby had no problem breathing, he was limp and unresponsive. The inertness continued, and on thorough examination, he was found to be a severely brain-damaged infant.

3. Deaf-blind.   Frank's mother had not known that she was pregnant until she consulted the doctor because of a slight rash she had. When the doctor informed her that a second baby was on the way, she and her husband were delighted. The rash was gone in a few days and was forgotten until Frank was born. The examination at birth revealed that the infant had cataracts in both eyes and a malformation of the heart valve. Frank's mother's rash had been rubella, and the virus had damaged the fetus in the early weeks of prenatal life. Frank's behavior in the first weeks and months was so unlike that of their first child. He seemed to prefer to be left alone rather than wanting to be held and loved. Eventually, surgery was required for the heart problem, and it was evident by then that he also had a serious hearing impairment.

Betty is an example of damage to the motor system, diagnosed as cerebral palsy, in addition to blindness. Paul had severe damage to a large part of the central nervous system and to the brain, which resulted in retarded physical and mental development. Frank had both his visual and auditory senses seriously impaired, and the heart condition posed a general health problem that limited his energy and stamina.

Blind or severely visually handicapped children like Betty, who have cerebral palsy, or additional motoric or anatomical problems such as spina bifida (an open spine), or degenerative conditions such as muscular dystrophy, may need a great deal of medical attention and perhaps even numerous surgical procedures. The normal developmental and learning processes will be interrupted even more dramatically than when there is only a visual problem. The severely brain-damaged child like Paul may have such extensive central nervous system or neurological damage that responses of any kind are difficult to elicit. Children like Frank, who have both visual and auditory loss and often a number of other impaired body systems as a result of maternal rubella, present perhaps the most complex problem in education. In such cases, being touched or handled may be unpleasant or painful; thus affectional interaction is not pleasurable or satisfying to the baby—something parents may find hard to understand or accept. Reciprocal rejection between parents and child limits both affective and psychomotor development and results in irreversible damage to any potential for cognitive growth.

Although each of the three groups just identified has some problems unique to the nature of the impairments, we will discuss the similarities and commonalities that apply to all of them. One great difficulty is in attempting to determine which of the impairments is of primary concern, and in some instances, who should assume the responsibility for educating these children. More important considerations may be: "What type of behavior is it possible to develop?" and "What kind of treatment is necessary to increase the probability that desirable behavior will be established?" (Ashcroft, 1966).

The total effect of multi-impairments may have little relation to the number of identified problems, and no two children with the same impairments have the same potential. Consequently, the approach to delineating the developmental and learning behaviors in affective, psychomotor, and cognitive domains must be individualized for each child.

Assessment, Diagnosis, and Interventions

When impairments occur in several body systems, it is difficult to predict developmental and learning potentials and to suggest specific prognoses. Evaluations should be made through interdisciplinary teams working in a variety of diagnostic settings over extended periods of time, both before and after the introduction of intervention procedures. Because medical persons are the most likely to see children with impairments first, their assessment can be specific in regard to which organs are impaired and the extent of the damage to the body system. However, because of all the other variables related to learning and development, the ultimate effect of the impairment cannot be predicted at an early age solely on the basis of the medical diagnosis. Doctors may be able to provide treatment or possibly surgical procedures or recommend therapeutic treatment that might help minimize the overwhelming long-term effects of the problem. In many instances, though, there may be little that medical personnel can do, especially in cases where there is damage to the central nervous system or the brain. In fact, it may be advisable to defer specific diagnoses when the long-term effects of such impairments may be undetermined. Many children with serious medical problems, some of whom may have required extensive surgery and hospitalization, have experienced few long-term developmental effects from the specific problem; whereas others with less extensive or less serious medical problems appear to have suffered greater and more widespread effects. Current information suggests benefits from giving more attention to special diets and vitamin therapy, but the long-term value of such treatments has not yet been determined.

Psychological and educational assessments and diagnoses are even more difficult and less certain; short-term, tentative predictions that can be reevaluated weekly, monthly, or as necessary appear to be the wisest approach. Diagnostic learning situations often show that some children need a continual assessment over a period of many months, if not several years, to determine with any degree of accuracy their potential for future development and to ascertain what interventions and prescriptive techniques should be used to achieve the best results. The reason for this long-term assessment is that, when damage to body systems is extensive, it may take many months to evoke responses to other human beings or to any object or environmental stimulus.

Once the child has indicated some awareness of the world around him, a breakthrough seems to occur, and carefully planned stimulation may indicate that the child can begin to develop some affective behaviors suggesting knowledge of a self and of others relating to that self. Structuring responses through various motor activities helps the child establish patterns of appropriate behaviors, and learning appears to begin at this point. Because of the complex difficulties of bringing a multi-impaired child to this point, short assessments and diagnoses in an office are of little value in planning educational experiences for the child. Specialists from many disciplines making assessments and diagnoses over a long period seem to provide the most valid information for teachers in planning learning experiences and developing individual prescriptive programs.

Teachers should be an integral part of the diagnostic team. They must be keen behavioral observers who can record and relate the child's functional level to a variety of developmental scales. Some teachers are capable of designing their own scales and checklists; others prefer to use those that are available. The important characteristic of any evaluative measure is that the sequence of behaviors be outlined from simple to more complex, and that each functional task be broken into small enough increments so that a realistic profile of each child emerges. Combined with other diagnostic and clinical data, teachers in cooperation with parents can determine the appropriate level of tasks with which to begin, in an attempt to increase the probability of success.

Learning Programs
and Prescriptive Teaching

Unlike more conventional educational programs, intervention strategies for multi-impaired children should be directed toward specific behavioral objectives for individual children. Often a one-to-one relationship between teacher and child is necessary to elicit the desired attention and functional behavior (Ashcroft, 1966). Every stage in the particular task or skill to be learned should be written in a step-by-step procedure so that there is consistency in approach and instructions. A structured program requires that each task or skill to be learned is analyzed carefully, defined in logical, sequential increments, and that success is achieved and rewarded promptly.

Even though the prescriptive program will be different for every child, certain basic educational curricula have been identified as most relevant (Best and Winn, 1968; Rogow, 1973; Talkington, 1972).

Human interactions and relationships: Pleasurable personal contacts; acceptance and trust of teachers, peers, and others; recognition of self and others as human beings.

Sensory awareness and stimulation: Exposure to sounds, odors, tastes, textures, and visual stimuli (if appropriate); discrimination and recognition of differences and likenesses.

Physical movement and activity: Body awareness and control (co-active movement with teacher); object manipulation and manual dexterity; exploratory movement in environment.

Self-care and daily living skills: Self-care skills of eating, dressing, and so forth; handling tools and materials; social play and interaction with others.

Language development and communication: Expression of personal needs and response to language (gesture, vocal, sign); word-object or word-action association; psychodrama, story telling, and role playing (records and tapes); following basic commands and instructions; meaningful language expression.

Work attitudes and habits development: Assigned work duties; personal and group responsibility; field trips on bus and public transportation.

Physical education and recreation: Tumbling, running, jumping, swimming, adapted games, arts and crafts.

Providing services for multi-impaired children requires creative and unorthodox systems involving many agencies and personnel from a variety of disciplines. When possible, such specialists as social workers, physical and occupational therapists, mental health workers, speech and language therapists, along with specially trained teachers and mobility instructors can cooperate to provide the broad spectrum of necessary services. Experimentation in a variety of settings can be effective and should be tried when appropriate to the community and state needs. Some possible settings are outlined below.

Home programs: For very young children, those in rural or sparsely populated areas. Teachers work in the home on a regular basis with parents teaching them how to work with children and developing specific prescriptive instructions.

Community agencies: Specialized agencies for blind, retarded, and/or cerebral palsied. These are day programs from two to six hours daily or several times a week for children with severe developmental lags.

Early childhood education for handicapped in public schools: For nursery- and kindergarten-level children. Less severely impaired children may be given intensive sensory and motor activities and personal and social skill development.

Day or residential programs: For specific groups such as "deaf-blind," "blind-disturbed," or "blind-retarded." State schools for the blind, community agencies, and public schools may service one or more of such designated groups when potential for continuing progress is indicated.

Self-contained classes in public schools: These are appropriate for those who are ready for specific skill development or who may be integrated eventually into work-study or other special programs within the total school system.

Institutional programs: Special teaching units in schools for retarded where children were institutionalized early in life and will probably remain there. A few may enter sheltered workshops or halfway houses.

Summary

Multi-impaired visually handicapped children are everywhere. New and daring innovations are being tried and severely damaged children, once thought hopeless, are beginning to function as human beings capable of learning far more than was ever imagined. Continued intensive efforts may bring forth even more advances during the next decade.

6

Tactual, Auditory, and Visual Development and Learning

In Chapter 3, we discussed the idea that affective development and the child's feelings about self and others are directly related to the quality and extent of human interaction. In Chapter 4, we developed the idea that psychomotor learning is facilitated by exploration, movement, and knowing how to control the body in order to respond purposefully in relationship to the environment and to objects within it.

Introduction to Sensory Learning

The development of cognitive ability—that is, knowing and thinking—involves the use of the senses, because nothing can be in the mind that has not first been received through the senses (Arnheim, 1969). What the child feels, hears, sees, tastes, and smells is internalized and stored as a model corresponding to the environment and determines what he knows about the world and about himself in relation to it (Bruner, 1966). Information coming through the senses must be received, interpreted, combined, and stored in the brain. The acquisition of language facilitates the integration of discrete sensory impressions to permit the learner to bring order to the material stored. Language also acts as a medium of exchange with others for clarifying and verifying sensory impressions. To be able to note the likenesses and differences between touch sensations, sights, sounds, tastes, and smells determines the later relationships developed between ideas. Integrating the myriad bits of concrete information received through the senses into a unified group of concepts about people and things provides the functional knowledge for thinking and talking about abstract ideas. The process of sorting, coding, and organizing sensory data and concepts to make all the characteristics and operational functions fit together is a complex mental task. Each child learns to do this in a unique manner, what Piaget (1973) called "a cognitive style of learning."

Seeking, selecting, ordering, and programming information evolves as a consistent, individual pattern that a child uses in his learning. This notion of unique learning patterns emphasizes the need for individualized instruction for maximal learning. Given this concept, parents and teachers should understand and accept each child's preferred learning strategies as appropriate for him (Keogh, 1973). Some theorists hypothesize that cognitive style may be well established by the age of three, but that it is amenable to alteration or modification for many years. Numerous studies have demonstrated that style affects learning success and achievement.

Learning progression.   Before trying to understand the visually handicapped child's specific problems in cognitive learning, we must first distinguish between the terms used to discuss sensory learning and the type and quality of information received through the different senses. Irrespective of the sense used to gather information, the term *discrimination* is used to refer to the ability to note the difference or likeness between objects or materials; this means the ability to distinguish whether what is being received is identical to, or distinct from, something else. *Recognition* means the ability to attach a name or label to a specific object or material; that is, to be able to identify what something is, what it does, the group to which it belongs, and its unique characteristics.

Discriminations and recognitions enable the child to develop perceptions about what he sees, hears, feels, smells, or tastes. That is, when he is able to give meaning to, understand, and interpret incoming information through the senses, then he is *perceiving* that information and is able to use it. Perception is an active process in that the learner is constantly seeking, attending to, and accepting information that is needed or desired and is ignoring sensory input that is useless or unnecessary (Foulke, 1968). Perceptual selection is determined by whether or not the received information fits with previously sorted information to give a different type or level of new understanding. Piaget refers to this process as "cognitive accommodation and assimilation."

Tactual-kinesthetic sense.   The tactual-kinesthetic senses are often referred to as the "skin" senses and may be given less significance than they actually deserve. Active involvement with the environment and with the objects in it is dependent on effective use of the tactual-kinesthetic sense, which is stimulated by mechanical, thermal, electrical, and chemical stimuli. The hands and other parts of the body can push, press, grasp, rub, and lift in order to get information. The fingertips, however, provide the most discrete (or distinct) impressions, the degree of accuracy exceeding even that of visual impressions (Fieandt, 1966). Using the muscles kinesthetically in movement or in handling objects or materials gives the most comprehensive and precise information. When one is unable to use the visual sense or when vision is severely impaired, information gained through the tactual-kinesthetic senses provides the individual with the most complete and reliable information.

Auditory sense.   The auditory sense functions through nerve endings that are deeply imbedded within the inner ear and surrounded by fluid. Stimulation through the sense of hearing is more difficult during the early months of life because the reception area for hearing is located deep within the center of the brain. Probably little usable information is available through the sense of hearing before three to six months of life (Fraiberg et al., 1969). Although the infant may show involuntary responses to sound, actual discrimination and recognition of sounds are not possible until several months after birth. When the human voice at very close range provides pleasurable auditory sounds, then the infant may begin to note other sounds. Soon he is able to begin to imitate sounds, especially the human voice. This imitation is an important process, since information fed to the brain through the auditory sense forms the basis for future language development and speech production.

Visual sense.   Because the visual sense provides a greater quantity and a more refined quality of information in a shorter period of time than does any other sense, vision is often thought to be the mediator between all other sensory information and is sometimes attributed with stabilizing the child's interaction with his world (Barraga, 1973). Most of what the young child learns incidentally (on his own and by himself) is learned through the visual sense. For this reason, the most efficient use of any existing visual capacity is critically important for visually handicapped children. When there is sufficient light to provide contrast between objects or to permit motion to be seen, there is potential for the child's using this visual information in meaningful ways.

Olfactory and gustatory senses.   The olfactory and gustatory senses react more readily to chemical qualities in the environment. The information received through the sense of smell may be very different from the information received through the sense of taste, even in response to the same stimulus. These two senses thus may give conflicting and confusing information, especially when they are simultaneously involved. The gustatory sense (without the use of olfaction) gives little specific information about flavor but gives a wider range of information about texture, contour, and size through the tip of the tongue and the sides of the mouth. The tip of the tongue is thought to have the most sensitive of all nerve endings in the body. Persons have even been able to read braille quite efficiently with the tip of the tongue.

The senses probably do not provide isolated information, but the extent and manner in which information received through a single sense can be transferred to another sense has not yet been determined. However, it may be that children are able to translate information through one sensory channel into another modality for storing and thinking (Buktenica, 1968). Regardless of the unsettled controversies regarding multisensory learning and intermodal transpositon of information, there is little question that every available sense needs to be used by children who have impairments in any one of the other senses. If the available senses are not developed, learning is likely to be fragmented and inaccurate.

Tactual Learning

The progression of sequential learning is similar for all of the senses. In visually handicapped children, however, greater attention may need to be given to each specific level and type of learning, since greater reliance is placed on senses other than vision. Let us use our example of Carl to illustrate each level within the sequence and the nature and type of learning in the development of the totally blind child.

Awareness and attention. Tactual-kinesthetic development begins with *awareness and attention* to differences in textures, temperatures, vibrating surfaces, and materials of varied consistencies. As Carl moves his hand along textures, presses against materials, and lifts objects, he begins to be aware that some are hard whereas others are soft, and some are rough whereas others are smooth. As he presses material such as clay and dough, he begins to understand that things he touches and handles have different consistencies. Putting his hands and body in water of different temperatures and moving himself and objects in water or in sand makes him aware that substances are not all alike nor do they behave in the same way.

As he touches objects that vibrate and those that do not, he learns that some give off stimulation and others do not. The blind child learns that he receives information from objects, and at the same time he is able to alter and adapt some objects through his tactual-kinesthetic handling, whereas he is unable to change others in any way.

Structure and shape. The second level of tactual-kinesthetic development relates to *knowledge of the basic structure and shape* of objects encountered. By moving his hand across objects, grasping and holding many shapes, and manipulating objects of various sizes, Carl acquires knowledge about contours and about variations in size and weight. Interaction for maximum information during this stage is best achieved through well-known objects that are part of the child's daily life, such as bars of soap, cups, plates, shoes, and socks. As Carl learns to discriminate between objects, it becomes appropriate to introduce language to teach recognition of specific objects. Cupping the hands around an object gives him a bit of gross information about it; moving his hands around and tracing the shape of an object gives him successive specific information about the object to enhance recognition by name.

The relation of parts to the whole.   Once Carl is able to recognize simple, everyday objects by name, the next level of tactual-kinesthetic development is possible. Whole objects that can be taken apart and put back together will help Carl learn *the relationship of parts to the whole.* At this stage, it is important for objects to be actual, three-dimensional things, such as toy cars that can be taken apart and put together, blocks that fit together, and household objects that have parts to be assembled. Putting lids on pans, keys in locks, and screwdrivers into heads of screws are examples of object manipulation relating parts to wholes.

Grouping objects according to texture is another appropriate learning experience at this stage. For example, Carl's mother may present to him all clothes that have the same texture, all silverware that is alike, blocks of the same texture, and buttons that feel alike. Additional learning should be focused on differences in size, length, and weight of objects. Manipulating objects increases skill in using the hands and in manual inspection. Concurrently, Carl becomes aware that he can exercise control over objects and make them work in specific ways; and through this handling, he begins to form concepts of the relationship of parts to wholes (Juurmaa, 1967). Practice in making finer and finer discriminations and maintaining the ability to recognize objects and parts of objects prepares the blind child for more complex tactual-kinesthetic learning related to academic work.

More complex manipulative experiences permit the child to develop for himself "tactual strategies" for fitting parts to each other and into a recognized whole. Carl developed such strategies because he was able to fit blocks to each other to complete a unified structure. Synthesizing tactual-kinesthetic impressions permits the child to make accommodations to new elements that he feels and rapidly to assimilate these in relation to the tactual information he already has.

Graphic representations.   Presenting *two-dimensional objects in graphic representation* is the next stage in tactual-kinesthetic development. Such representations may be made by string or wire, with a tracing wheel or stylus, on foil, plastic, or paper. The graphic representation of a real object may bear little tactual resemblance to the known object, and what is perceived may not fit with previously stored information. The spatial perspective in a graphic representation is often quite unlike the spatial perspectives perceived by handling. Selecting simple structural patterns such as geometric forms, available to be handled and represented in two dimensions, permits the child gradually to gain successive tactual impressions, and as his fingertips and muscles move in certain patterns, he learns to associate the real object and the one represented. For example, once a child easily recognizes round objects or forms, then various sizes of roundness may be graphically represented for the child to examine. Carl was not old enough to have reached this stage, but gradually increasing the experiences to include many shapes and structural forms will provide the basic experiences necessary for later learning (Barraga, Dorward, and Ford, 1973).

Such graphic representations as raised lines, curves, simple geometric forms, and object outlines of very well-known things should be introduced slowly. It is important to provide only one piece of information at a time. As that basic information is interpreted, then one additional element may be added in successive graphic representation. For example, if one is going to prepare graphic material for the child to tactually perceive a human figure, the stick portion representing the body and the child's understanding this relationship to the straight postural position of the body could be the first step. Adding a circle for the head would be the next step; then adding straight lines to represent arms and legs could be associated to the lines of the body and the roundness of the head. Adding lines to represent fingers and toes could complete the figure. In contrast, giving the entire graphic representation at one time could be very confusing and has been called "tactual noise" (Hammill and Crandell, 1968).

Also appropriate at this time is to teach the child to make his own graphic drawings. As he makes a line with a tracing wheel or with a tool on a piece of aluminum foil or on a raised-line drawing board, the child begins to realize how his body is moving in order to make certain lines or forms. Realizing that he is making pictures that he can "see" with his own hands is exciting and provides motivation to examine everything on paper or in books that is tactually perceivable. This desire and skill prepare him for interpreting abstract tactual representations.

Braille symbols.   The highest level of tactual-kinesthetic development is discrimination and recognition of symbols in the form of braille characters that represent letters, words, and stories of the child's own experiences. Symbol recognition through the visual sense requires a high level of visual coding and association, but the tactual discrimination and recognition of symbols in the form of braille characters is an even more abstract level of perceptual-cognitive association. The totally blind child must not only recognize the symbols tactually (which in itself is a high-order task), but he must also interpret their meanings in relation to other surrounding braille characters and also in the context of the material he is reading. This places a burden on tactual-kinesthetic memory and requires immediate decision making on the part of the child in relation to recognition, memory, association, and interpretation (Henderson, 1973).

Returning to Carl and his manipulative experiences, if his early preschool experiences continue to provide a wide variety of tactual-kinesthetic exposure and manipulation, then his readiness for academic learning through reading would be more advanced than that of a child who did not have preschool experiences that provided the appropriate development in tactual-kinesthetic learning. In instances in which the blind child has not had complete tactual-kinesthetic development before entering educational programs, the teacher's role may be quite different from that normally expected in a school setting, since braille reading would have to be deferred. The appropriate experiences for developing to the refined stage of symbol recognition would need to become part of the child's readiness curriculum, and in some rare instances, could require several years before the child were ready to begin more formal types of academic skills such as reading.

The tactual reading process is more complex than the visual reading process because of the numerous braille characters (sixty-three possible dot combinations in the six-dot braille cell) and because of the contractions used in embossed material in the abbreviated Grade 2 braille. Many braille symbols have multiple uses, and the interpretation of their meaning depends on their relationship to other characters, their position in the cell, and the initial, medial, or final position within the word or sentence. Braille symbols representing the same letter or word may be different within a single sentence; hence, decision making in braille reading requires a high level of ability in cognitive abstraction. Only those children who have achieved the mental flexibility and processing necessary for this task can be efficient in tactual reading as a primary means of learning (Henderson, 1973). Children who are functioning below average mentally are not likely to learn to read using braille, unless special materials are prepared. The braille symbols should be introduced gradually: at first, only those standing for a single letter are appropriate; later, symbols representing whole words could be incorporated. Thorough understanding and recognition of each group of symbols is imperative before adding a more complex group.

For a moment, let us consider the need for tactual-kinesthetic learning in a low-vision child such as Lucy. Even though some visual capacity is present, and she has begun to use it early in life, there is still need to give the same attention to her tactual-kinesthetic development as was necessary for Carl. Touching and feeling objects will help clarify and support the unclear images she receives visually. Maximum tactual-kinesthetic development in the low-vision child will unify all sensory input and enable the child to form more stable concepts.

Thinking back to Dora and Keith, who experienced visual loss after their early developmental years, we see differences in tactual-kinesthetic development. In Dora's case, vision was limited but was still her primary information-gathering sense organ. She probably used her tactual sense to a limited degree, and as she experienced more and more loss of vision, she possibly began to rely unconsciously on touch and feel to supplement her learning. The use of the two senses, simultaneously or alternately, probably enabled her to develop and refine her perceptions of touch and movement with comparative ease and efficiency. Nevertheless, when children experience progressive visual loss, parents and teachers must concentrate specifically on tactual development by providing a wide range of tactual experiences, until the child feels secure and demonstrates proficiency in tactual discrimination and recognition.

When a child or youth such as Keith has been blinded suddenly, the transfer to tactual learning is far more difficult and is likely to take a much longer time. Although much incidental tactual and kinesthetic perception has occurred, because of his former ability to use the dominant visual sense, Keith has not consciously attended to these perceptions since he had little need to do so. For these reasons, a newly blinded child or youth will need the same intensive program in tactual perceptual development as would be required for a totally blind infant. Associations will be easier and concepts more readily developed by concentrating on the store of visual memories; mental imagery will become a composite of visual and tactual perceptions and eventual concepts. The sensitivity of tactual receptors will need to be sharpened through continually expanded experiences focused on tactual discrimination and recognition of concrete objects and two-dimensional graphic representations before introducing braille characters, which require very fine tactual discrimination. Materials are available for blinded youth and adults who need a gradual exposure to the more easily recognized braille symbols.

Auditory Development and Learning

There is a frequent tendency to think that the ears of a blind person are comparable to the eyes of a sighted person for providing information. There is some truth to this, but one must exercise caution in accepting this idea without qualification. Because of the nature of the auditory sense and the continuous presence of inescapable sound in the environment, the human being has little physical control over auditory input but instead must learn to exercise mental control—*selective perception.* This "masking" of sound occurs through a selective process, at first unconsciously and then later according to the meaningfulness of the sound to the individual. The mere presence of sound does not necessarily mean that the individual listens to or hears it.

While sound and auditory input are a primary source of contact with the environment for visually limited children, excessive auditory stimulation of meaningless sounds may evoke verbal repetition, or echolalic responses, to sound and actually inhibit the use of auditory input as a means of learning. Mere auditory stimulation must not be confused with meaningful auditory input translatable into learning experiences. Therefore, parents and teachers should direct specific attention to the sequence in auditory development in visually handicapped children, the relationship of speech and language development to auditory development, the use of hearing as a primary learning medium, the development of efficient listening skills, and the relation of auditory development to language development as instruments for thinking.

The sequential pattern for the formation of auditory perceptions and concepts is similar to that of tactual-kinesthetic development and visual development, although the appropriate application of these sequential ideas to the visually handicapped child is clearly different for hearing than for touching.

Environmental sounds.   The first level of learning through the sense of hearing is that of *awareness and attention* to specific environmental sounds. The infant may be both soothed and startled by sounds, whereas many noises appear to have little effect on the very young baby. Part of the reason for this fact is that only sounds of great intensity, either in volume or pitch, penetrate through the infant's auditory receptive system, which is actually a built-in protective device since the infant has not yet learned to mask confusing or disturbing sounds.

To bring soothing sound into awareness, the young visually handicapped child should have the opportunity to hear many pleasing and comforting sounds such as soft music and the human voice. These sounds create in the infant an unconscious awareness and attachment to the environment, in addition to conveying affective feelings of warmth and comfort. Even in a young infant, before specific sounds are attended to, sound from the human voice provides a feeling of communication and attachment, probably substituting for facial expressions and gestures, which do not exist for the totally blind child. Without exposure to the human voice in the first few months of life, the totally blind child may feel as if he were living in total isolation (Fraiberg et al., 1969). Continual and appropriate vocal stimulation in the early months may help the blind child learn to use this auditory contact in much the same way that the sighted child uses eye movement to follow the actions of those around him. Placing bells or other pleasant noises on objects the infant touches or on another person helps to stabilize the idea that there are many sounds within his environment. In the early months, it is appropriate to urge the infant to listen to specific pleasant sounds as he is moved about by someone else.

Specific sounds.   Although the infant who is blind may show awareness of sound and attend to a few specific sounds, the second level of development—*response to specific sounds*—probably does not occur before approximately four to six months of age (Fraiberg et al., 1969). Responses to specific sounds may be in the form of smiling, turning the head, listening intently and silently, and later attempting to imitate vocally. This behavior suggests that the child is beginning to maintain contact with specific sounds and localize the source of the sound. Turning the head in response to specific sounds suggests that "listening to hear" (Piaget, 1973) is the intent; and at this stage, ear-hand coordination (again, comparable to eye-hand coordination in the sighted child) is possible. The manipulation of objects simply to hear sound may be observed, indicating the beginning of autonomy in knowledge that a certain hand action may produce a particular sound. Knowledge that sound can be associated with an object implies that the baby can be taught to reach for sound, such as in searching for a toy or moving toward an appealing sound.

Sound discrimination.   Discrimination between familiar household and outdoor sounds, voices, and musical tones is the next level in auditory development for the visually handicapped child. By this time, the baby may move in relation to household sounds to find the source of the sound. Parents should encourage this activity and permit the child to tactually explore sounds to which he gives attention and can localize. This is also the appropriate time to name the sources of the sounds to develop the knowledge that sounds come from different things in the home and to permit the child to associate sounds with the things he touches. By noting the differences in environmental sounds and voices, the child is learning to connect his own actions and those of others with specific sounds. As these associations become more frequent and refined, he may be able to make discoveries for himself by following sounds and moving to them.

Naming the source of the sound and encouraging vocal mimicking is quite important. Such guidance in auditory development permits the child to organize his own behavior as it relates to a specific goal or purpose in his movement in relation to sound. For example, the severely visually handicapped child may begin to recognize people by the differences in their voices or their footsteps, and may actually associate the footsteps or voices with anticipation of the event to occur. For example, one blind child, upon hearing her father's footsteps, learned to say the first meaningful words, "Go-car." This came about from the fact that when the father arrived each day, the child was taken for a ride in the car. Very shortly, she had learned to associate the sound of the father's footsteps with the anticipation of going for a drive.

At this level of development, sound begins to replace vision for perceiving distance relationships and may also serve as a primary motivation for movement as the child is learning to walk. Movement in relation to sound may also provide (unconsciously perhaps) incidental development in the use of sound echoes to indicate the presence of objects. The level of sound as the child approaches an object becomes a referent for distance in addition to guiding direction in movement. The greater the range and variety of sound sources toward which the child can move and also touch, the more rapidly his development in discrimination and familiarity will proceed, and the more stable the base for interpreting sound.

Sound recognition and association.   As words begin to have meaning to the child, the next level of auditory development—*recognition of sounds related to specific words and connected speech*—is possible. Just as the child is learning that objects have names, he may learn also that sounds have specific words associated with them and that his own actions have words to describe them. To assist him in this process of recognition and association, parents should talk about the child's movements and actions, interpret in words for him what is happening when he responds to certain "noise-makers," and clearly differentiate between the sounds of words. There is some indication that imitative speech in relation to auditory input comes about more rapidly in the visually handicapped child than in the sighted child. This is probably related to the fact that without the full use of the visual sense, attending to auditory input develops acuity and a greater sensitivity to sound. There is no indication that visually handicapped children have any greater capacity for auditory perception than do sighted children, but their constant use and heavy reliance on the auditory sense permits development to proceed rapidly.

Remember that it is important when a child responds to sound to give him the opportunity to interpret it fully by touching its source whenever possible, or by having the sound interpreted to him through words. Talking to a visually handicapped child as he moves and plays is more important than talking to a sighted child, since the only way the visually handicapped child can interpret the meaning of his own actions is through the help of others who talk to him, providing meaning through auditory input. As mentioned earlier, passive auditory stimulation from radio or television without meaningful verbal discourse with adults often results in echolalic speech, or verbalizations that have no real meaning for the child and do not contribute to cognitive development. Playing word games and reading nursery rhymes while holding or playing with the child strengthen sound association and memory.

Interpreting verbal instructions.   Recognition of voices and understanding words and directions, the next level of auditory perceptual development, is the stage when visually handicapped children may be taught selective listening. They have achieved the ability to mask out irrelevant or meaningless sounds and attend to musical themes, speech that provides directions and instructions, and they may now begin to formulate their own speech for feedback to themselves and to others. Through an auditory feedback process, the adult will recognize discrepancies in meaning and inaccuracies that have occurred because the child hears without being able to see. For example, adults can play games that focus on identifying voices of specific people by questioning, "Who is that?" Another aid is to make tape recordings of environmental and household sounds and ask the child to talk about what he is hearing as he listens to the recording.

Translating vocal instructions into purposeful actions is one of the highest levels of auditory perceptual processing, especially in a young child. Given the proper opportunity to develop through the previously mentioned stages, the child should be able to respond and carry out actions according to instructions given to him.

A young child who is unable to do this should be given greater attention to determine whether he understands the meanings of the words he hears in relation to his own movement and actions. Unless the child can translate auditory input into meaningful options or associations that he can use, there is little indication that auditory input is relating to cognitive development. For the visually handicapped child, the cognitive translation of auditory language provides mental stimulation that may be equivalent to the sighted child's motivation through visual perceptual skills. The child forms action images in relation to spoken language, and this imagery creates a basis for recall and for higher-level abstract thinking when the words are no longer heard. For example, when instructions are given to move the body to a specific position or to walk in a particular pattern, the child has to think about what he has heard and translate this into his body actions. Later, when he hears the same or similar instructions, he remembers movement pattern to which he can relate. Translating what is heard into personal meaning may stimulate searching for meaning in other spoken messages.

Auditory skills and listening in learning. Once the visually handicapped child enters school, one of his primary channels for learning will be hearing. Consequently, achieving the highest level of auditory processing and listening efficiency is essential for further cognitive development. Paying attention to the sequence in auditory development and perception just outlined will avoid the mistaken assumption that simply because the child has the capacity to hear, he is able to use his listening efficiently for academic learning. Processing through the auditory sense without the preparatory perceptual skills is a practically impossible task.

Acquiring information tactually through reading braille is a slow process. As the child progresses through school, he may realize that he has developed his listening skills to the extent that auditory input for learning is often presented at a much slower rate than his brain is capable of processing. For this reason, experiments in production and reception of "speeded" speech have been conducted (Foulke, 1968; Nolan, 1966; Tuttle, 1971). As visually handicapped youth reach junior and senior high school, reliance on listening as a primary means of learning reaches its peak; and any future pursuit in higher education will require almost total reliance on listening for learning. Therefore, researchers are concentrating on refining aural study systems for visually handicapped students (Brothers, 1971; Nolan and Morris, 1967).

Cognitive Development

Piaget suggests that there are many object classes that the blind child cannot act on perceptually (through vision or hearing or motorically) and must simply know in terms of the symbolic auditory language. This may present a problem referred to as "verbalism"—that is, using words without understanding their meaning. Studies of cognitive development in blind children (Higgins, 1973; Tobin, 1972; Witkin, Oltman, Chase, and Friedman, 1971) have indicated some lag in abstract thinking and in the meaningful use of language without the performance of concrete operations or having available concrete materials. Boldt (1970) found that cognitive development proceeded along similar lines in visually handicapped children; but their ability to handle auditory material suffered a tremendous lag until about the age of sixteen or eighteen, which is several years behind that of sighted children. This exemplifies the fact that simply auditory processing and verbalizing appropriate words does not mean necessarily that the words are completely understood cognitively. Numerous studies have found that blind children are less able to define the meaning of vocabulary words than are their sighted peers of comparable age and intellectual ability. A broad generalization suggests that blind children may know and use a word but are unable to express a cause-effect relationship, possibly because of the lack of a mental image to use as a referent (Stephens, 1972).

It appears that without vision, many concepts cannot be fully developed without carefully planned teaching strategies to counterbalance the perceptive privation. A comprehensive study of cognitive development in congenitally blind children is currently being completed, and a subsequent plan for remediation of identified deficits is projected. More specific information may be available in the near future.

Other studies have shown a somewhat superior ability in totally blind youth to sustain auditory attention and to process material auditorially. Therefore, no general conclusions would be applicable to all blind children; the individual characteristics of each child must be considered in relation to his previous background and experience. The evidence presented in the picture of Carl suggests that his auditory perceptual abilities were in keeping with his level of development, as demonstrated by his awareness of footsteps indicating the arrival of someone, his ability to understand verbal instructions and to act accordingly, and his ability to localize sound sources and use them in efficient movement in his familiar surroundings. When Carl reaches school age, there is good reason to believe that his auditory perceptual abilities and listening skills will have developed to a level that will permit him to expand and refine them for use in mobility training and as one of his primary means of learning to read.

Lucy, who has questionable visual ability, will need as careful attention to auditory perceptual development as for tactual-kinesthetic development. Because of the probability of limited vision throughout her school years, she will need to use auditory learning as one of her supplemental, if not her primary, senses for learning. Auditory perception and careful listening may assist her in clarifying the incomplete or blurred visual impressions she receives. Obviously, her low vision will limit or preclude the use of vision as a distance sense, and Lucy will be required to rely on audition as her distance sense. Sound localization will be her major safety clue in movement and travel outside the home.

Dora, because of her spontaneous adjustment to the gradual loss of sight, has no doubt already begun to use sound as a key referent in her environmental interactions. As visual loss continues, her parents and teachers should direct her toward refining auditory localization skills and listening skills to help her bridge the transfer from visual learning to tactual learning. She must be taught to use some caution in movement so that she may learn to be sensitive to her own safety.

Efficient braille reading will develop slowly for Dora, during which time she will rely heavily on listening and auditory learning as she perfects her skills. In her educational program, she will probably use both tactual and auditory learning to complement each other and to enable her to continue in her achievements in schoolwork and related activities.

Because of his sudden loss of sight, Keith will rely strongly on auditory cues almost immediately. However, his parents and teachers should carefully structure a programmatic approach to developing auditory perceptual abilities to facilitate his actions and to encourage and permit his continued participation in social activities and in academic learning. Tactual learning and braille reading will be very slow at first, and Keith will rely almost exclusively on auditory learning and listening as his primary means of keeping up in school. Although interpreting what he hears in school-related material will be of first-order importance, refining his auditory sensitivity and auditory perceptions in environmental tasks should not be overlooked. Following a developmental sequence from the lowest level to the more complex should be adhered to, until he has begun to use listening as an efficient means of continuing his cognitive development.

There is no immediate transfer from the use of one sense to another sense upon the loss of the dominant sense of vision. Assuming that this occurs can be misleading and constitute a serious disservice to the child, unless he is assisted in developing proficiency in auditory processing.

Visual Development and Learning

Since approximately seventy-five to eighty percent of all school-age visually handicapped children have some usable vision and will either be low-vision children or visually limited children, of major importance is developing maximum visual perceptual ability in visually handicapped children. The past tendency to equate the extent of visual impairment with the limitation in seeing imposed on the individual has been found to have no basis in reality. Neither does the assumption that visual acuity has any relationship to the capacity for visual development or for actual visual functioning (Faye, 1970). Another erroneous assumption has been that children with impaired vision should be protected from eye strain, and that using the eyes could in some way damage the remaining vision. Faye again suggests that, "Residual vision should be used to the maximum capacity of the child," which from a perceptual and learning point of view means that the more the child looks and uses his vision, the more efficiently he will be able to function visually.

Just as hearing is not related only to the structure of the ear, vision is not related only to the structure and function of the eyes but involves many parts of the eyes as well as other body systems. The diagram below identifies the components of the total visual system and the particular function of each in relation to the total process of visual interpretation. The physiological struc-

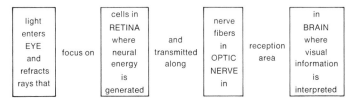

tures in the eye, such as the pupil and lens, facilitate or impede the rays of light from reaching the sensitive retinal cells. The location and spread of the activated cells help determine the strength of the burst of energy sent along the optic nerve to the brain, where the person interprets the electrical charges as visual information and relates it to messages received from the other senses.

Visual skills.   Such skills as fixation, tracking, focus, accommodation, and convergence are achieved by the majority of children with normal vision in their day-to-day functioning. However, the child with a visual impairment may have difficulty in developing these skills, dependent on the type as well as the severity of the impairment. When very little light can enter the eye or reach the nerve centers in the retina, muscular control may be difficult to develop and assistance, guidance, and even training may be necessary to permit the child to use his eyes with the highest possible degree of skill. Perfecting or refining such skills will enhance the child's visual functioning, since it will be much easier for him to receive visual impressions. As more and more visual stimulation occurs, he will naturally begin to use his eyes with greater efficiency.

Although skillful use of the eyes may not, by itself, enhance visual learning, it certainly increases the possibility of perceptual development through the visual sense. Of course, actual seeing cannot occur until messages transmitted through the eyes are received in the brain and there interpreted. Even when visual information is blurred, distorted, or incomplete, as long as the brain is able to combine the images with auditory and other sensory information, the person can use vision as a contributing sense in his cognitive development.

Numerous medical specialists and educational researchers have shown that poor vision does not necessarily cause poor learning—what the brain is able to do with the visual information it receives determines how well the person will be able to function visually (Bateman and Weatherall, 1967; Faye, 1970).

Visual perceptual development. Just as was the case in tactual and auditory development and learning, the use of the visual sense follows a progressive sequence, from a perceptual and learning point of view. The first level is that of *awareness,* which is encouraged by providing stimulating sights and calling attention to things on which to focus. Objects having a definite contour and that are brightly colored or reflect light easily should be brought close to the child, then moved away a distance to teach him to fixate on something to see and learn to move his eyes in relation to objects. These objects should be turned in various ways and introduced from the sides and from the front, so that the child learns to look from various angles. As the child is taken around the room or outside, he should be brought close to things and asked to touch them or have his hand reach out to them, to begin the coordination of eye-hand movements. Skill in using the eye muscles is brought under control, fixating is stabilized, and focusing the two eyes together is encouraged (if there is visual capacity in both) by consistently guiding the child, urging him to look, and providing stimuli that he may be able to see. A light source, such as a flashlight or other moving light, is good stimulation for helping the child to hold his eyes steady and look at a specific thing. As always, what he sees should be talked about so that words begin to be associated with the fact that there is something to see.

Form perception is the next stage in the developmental process. As the baby begins to move about, he should have the opportunity to encounter objects of many different forms, both large and small. As language begins to develop, the names of objects should be introduced, and their specific qualities such as curves, lines, corners, and points should be emphasized. At this level, parents should present many sizes of the same brightly colored object in addition to carefully selected toys. The primary concern at this stage is to provide contrast between objects and backgrounds to facilitate looking and reaching. Sometimes it is appropriate to place objects within a small area around the baby to encourage him to look and reach for those he finds interesting. As soon as crawling and walking begin, parents should call attention to large objects within the environment to make the child aware of them visually and of the form they present. Although an infant may not be able to see them except in gross form at this stage, he will learn to move his body in relation to stationary objects. Also, objects that move in front and to the side of the child should be part of this early stimulation to make him realize that there are things to see in many different directions.

As soon as the child has shown an awareness of objects, has begun to notice forms within the environment, and has demonstrated an ability to move in relation to them, the child's parents and teachers can concentrate on the next stage of development—*form perception of objects represented in pictures and other visual displays.* Since most visually handicapped children and almost all low-vision children see things at a near point with much greater clarity than at a distance, looking at pictures, books, and magazines should be a pleasurable and motivating activity. The pictures of objects should be simple at first and probably in solid colors, either black on white or other bright colors against contrasting backgrounds. At the beginning, these pictures should be medium in size and then gradually reduced as the child is still able to see them.

As soon as he is pointing to and naming simple solid pictures, the child may be introduced to simple outline pictures that have distinct forms and unique shapes. Only later should pictures of objects with detail be introduced, since too much detail is confusing and distracting to children who have severe visual limitations. The child's recognition of familiar objects in represented form should be accompanied, when appropriate, by the actual object for the child to handle, compare, and associate with the picture of the object. Objects represented in pictures should be shown from different perspectives to include aspects of spatial position and arrangement into the perceptual task.

By the time the child is approximately three years old, has come to enjoy looking at pictures of objects in books, and has begun to move about by using his sense of vision, he is ready to be introduced to visual materials at the next level—*environmental scenes, discrimination and recognition of pictorial figures, or depictions of action.* It is important to call attention to how the images differ from each other for the child to learn to pick out the differences between objects or persons. The child may be asked to imitate with his own body simple stick figures representing body actions. Later he should be able to look at pictures of certain situations and talk about what is occurring in the pictures. Looking at a series of pictures showing familiar objects or actions provides an opportunity for visual concept development in relation to size, near and distance perspectives, and the differences in the way things look from changed positions.

At the same time, the child's movement in larger space and in relation to adults and other children should be emphasized. He may be taught to imitate others' body actions through vision, supported by an adult's actually manipulating the child's body to help him clarify the nature of the action and his own body's position. Such activity is important for the visually limited child's future efficiency in seeking out knowledge for himself for his future independent movement in the environment.

Such activities as visual sorting, grouping, and categorizing should be part of the visually limited child's play at this stage. He may group or sort according to color, size, length, or the use or sequence of events. Clothing, kitchen utensils, thread and buttons, along with such toys as blocks, dolls, cars, and beads are appropriate materials to use. These sorting and grouping tasks should be carried out according to the verbal instructions of an adult, who can also identify and correct inaccuracies.

Eye-hand coordination, often difficult for low-vision and visually limited children, can be fostered by frequent opportunities to mark or draw with felt-tipped pens, large crayons, and paint brushes. Making pictures with colored yarn or scraps of colored paper is another good activity. Talking about and interpreting what is being done is important for the child.

A still higher level of visual perceptual development is *visual memory, visual closure, visual unification, and visual organization.* This aspect of visual development assumes the ability to hold in memory visual images and to be able to organize them in the mind so as to anticipate the whole when only partial segments of the whole are visible. To demonstrate this level of visual development, the child should be able to work with puzzles to take them apart, but more significantly, to be able to fit the pieces together again in relation to the picture of the whole which he holds in his mind. This facet of visual functioning is important for all preschool children but is especially so for the visually handicapped child with usable vision, since he will be required to recognize many things when he can see only parts of them. This exercise is designed to help him make more accurate predictions about what he is seeing. Many games should be played with children who have limited vision in discriminating missing portions and putting together simple and subsequently more complex puzzles. Guessing games about what he is seeing visually are another good device.

The stability of visual skills and self-assurance in the ability to use limited vision effectively prior to attempting more abstract types of visual activities, such as the *discrimination and recognition of letters and words,* are essential for the development of children with limited vision. If a broad background of experiences and many aspects of visual perceptual development are not fully realized, the visually limited child will not be ready to be introduced to abstract material such as print reading. In many instances, a child was thought unable to read because he was unable to see the letters or words; in reality, he may have been well able to see the letters and words, but his visual perceptual development was so incomplete that he lacked the basic frames of reference and flexible skills required to make associations to real objects and events within the environment.

When visually limited children, especially those who have very low vision, enter school, it is often necessary to spend a long period of time in visual perceptual development as a part of readiness before attempting to introduce visual reading material. The use of the visual sense in severely visually handicapped children was long neglected, and only recently has using any small amount of existing vision been stressed as a means of learning and a facilitator for higher levels of cognitive development. This new emphasis has been the impetus for several studies and finally a concerted effort to teach all children with any degree of visual capability to learn to use it for all learning purposes, even though the primary learning for academic success may not be achieved through use of vision (Barraga, 1964, 1970).

Lucy, whose parents were told that it was impossible to tell at an early age to what extent her visual capabilities might develop, is an example of a low-vision child who will probably need a long period of readiness in visual activities designed specifically to acquaint her with print symbols and enable her to relate these to visual concepts that she may have experienced in her preschool years. However, these activities will need to be stabilized and associated very gradually as she learns to use her vision for acquiring information in school.

Since Dora is gradually losing her vision, she will need help and guidance in continuing to retain her visual imagery and interpreting things that she can no longer see clearly, although she has retained visual memories of these objects with which to associate. Children who are losing vision will retain functioning for a much longer period if they are encouraged to use their vision and helped to interpret and make decisions about the unclear visual information they receive.

Even when all senses are intact, children seem to use different senses in varying degrees and for their own purposes. Some children with rather good vision look very little, whereas others with very limited vision look quite intently. However, cognitive development follows a more stable pattern with the use of all available senses; and only when all senses are used to their maximum capability will learning and cognitive development reach the optimum for each child. Whether the child is totally blind, has very low vision, or is only visually limited, he needs the opportunity to explore the use of all his senses and to develop for himself the unique styles of learning that give the greatest quantity and the highest quality of usable information for cognitive development.

Summary

In recent years, education has focused greater attention on the role of the senses in learning and cognitive development for all children, and especially for children who are visually handicapped. Every child with a visual impairment needs to be encouraged in his early years and perhaps throughout his school years to support and confirm the information he is receiving and to search out additional information through the use of his tactual sense. The tactual sense keeps the child in direct contact with the concrete world and provides a range of information that may not be available to him visually, and that lacks clarity and precision when experienced only through his sense of hearing.

All visually handicapped children must learn to rely heavily on auditory input as a primary means of alerting them to what may be seen or of keeping them in contact with distance information that will never be available to them visually. For congenitally totally blind children, auditory information will be their primary guide to movement, even in familiar environments, and later will provide cues for safe movement in new environments and eventually in independent travel. Similarly, the youth who has lost vision at a later stage will need to develop auditory sensitivities to be alerted to every sound emanating from the environment and to use sound clues as a valuable means of associating previously seen information with what now can only be heard.

7   Differential Programming and Educational Media

Controversies need not always be viewed as negative; at times they may act as instigators for reformed action and progress. This appears to have been true in the education of visually handicapped children in the past twenty-five years. Prior to 1950, discussions and arguments centered on such things as what materials to use (braille codes, large type), the proper application of educational equipment and gadgetry (arithmetic slates), and the specific methodologies appropriate for "blind children" (save sight by not using it). These issues no doubt seemed important at the time, especially to a small group of teachers and administrators associated primarily with residential schools. However, as broader educational issues came into perspective and public school programs began to assume some responsibility for teaching visually handicapped children, the focus shifted to the children themselves as learners and to new and different ways for these children to acquire the same information available to children with better vision.

Educators have come to realize that there is no single answer that prescribes the way all children ought to be taught nor a single medium or piece of equipment that is appropriate for all visually handicapped children. This recognition has probably been the primary impetus for innovative educational planning and programming during recent years. There are now a multitude of approaches rather than one method for all, many possible settings for the child's educational experience, and a diversity of equipment and materials to facilitate learning for the visually handicapped.

Merely substituting tactual, auditory, or enlarged visual material and different equipment for teaching the visually handicapped is no longer an accepted model to which educators are bound. Because each child has different learning characteristics, an individual means of acquiring information, and other variables associated with learning, programs for the visually handicapped must be planned specifically according to each child's level of functioning and according to the best approach to enhance learning for effective daily living.

**Educational Settings and
Services**

Visually handicapped children today are being served in a large number
of educational settings. The choice of setting is usually related to the availability of facilities, the child's needs at a particular stage of development, and other
considerations related to each family. Community nursery school programs
serve visually handicapped children who are able to function without too much
individual assistance within a group of sighted children. Visually limited children and a few low-vision children may adapt well to such a setting. Socialization and development of many affective characteristics that contribute to the
child's personal, emotional, and social development can be gained through
association with normally seeing children.

Special nursery schools, either private or attached to community agencies,
may be more appropriate for severely visually handicapped children who may
be slower in their development, and also for totally blind children, who need
more specialized attention and can learn to function more easily in a group
of children having similar psychomotor limitations and who learn primarily
through the senses of touch and hearing. Some severely visually handicapped
and totally blind children develop rapidly and may be included in nursery
programs with sighted children when their movement skills and their self-
directive learning strategies permit them to participate within the total group.
Very few residential educational programs are available to children under the
age of four or five years.

The value of complete parental involvement in any early educational
program cannot be overemphasized. Parents should be included as part of the
educational team in designing experiences, delivering the services, and evaluating their children's progress. Teachers and preschool counselors provide information, support, and guidance to parents. In addition, interaction and participation with parents of other visually handicapped children can have unlimited
merit for some parents. Most of the special nursery schools and regional and
state preschool programs encourage and provide leadership for parent groups
to create an understanding of the things their children are, or should be,
learning; therefore, the likelihood of the child's making progress is increased
when socialization and educational experiences are continued in the home and
neighborhood.

The current emphasis on kindergarten and early childhood education for
all children, and especially the legislative provisions for early childhood education programs for the handicapped, have opened the way for many children
and their families to participate in preschool activities that would not previously have been available because of geographic location or the lack of funds
for establishing such programs. Programs for kindergarten and early childhood education for the handicapped are found in community agencies and
often as part of public school programs. In many instances, residential schools

have developed programs for children who live in remote rural areas where specialized personnel are not available to work with them and their parents, or for those who need a residential program due to family circumstances. The objective of most of these programs is to develop learning readiness for children to pursue academic programs. Children who have additional impairments that contribute to pronounced lags in development and readiness may need to continue readiness programs in segregated settings for a longer time, eventually being placed in vocational programs that put greater emphasis on practical living than on academic learning.

Children like Carl and Lucy will probably develop the necessary learning skills and move into regular school programs with little difficulty. Recent studies (Hull, 1973) indicate that when low-vision children are given special training in visual development at kindergarten levels, they are able to move into regular school programs and perform as competently as their seeing peers. Although this may not be true for all low-vision children, the idea is worth considering. All severely visually handicapped children should be given the opportunity to experience the specialized learning experiences available through kindergarten and early childhood educational programs.

The attitude adopted nearly twenty years ago (Abel, 1959)—advocating that no one educational setting is the most appropriate for all visually handicapped children, and that a diversity of educational settings is desirable to meet the needs of children and their families—is still valid. The acceptance of this idea has resulted in programs' expanding into a variety of settings during the elementary and secondary school years. At the present time, however, between sixty and sixty-five percent of school-age visually handicapped children receive services within their home communities and, in most cases, within public school settings.

Organizational programming and services differ from community to community and from state to state. Ideally, program patterns should be determined by the needs of the children to be served, even though this is neither always possible nor is it the primary consideration. Organizational patterns are often based on the availability of personnel, the attitudes of individual school districts, and administrative expediency, rather than on an objective appraisal of the needs of children to be served.

Identifying those needing services.   Even before nursery or kindergarten age, totally blind children and most of those with severe visual impairment will have been identified by parents if not diagnosed by specialists. However, many visually limited children (having less severe impairments) may never have been examined to determine the clarity of their vision at both near and far distances or whether they see equally well with both eyes. A trend in recent years has been to stress the need for screening all young children for visual problems as soon as they are able to respond cooperatively to visual charts. The majority of near-sighted children can be identified easily even in preschool years by the standard Snellen eyechart with E symbols of different sizes and arranged in different positions. The National Society for the Prevention of Blindness sponsors screening programs throughout the country. Strabismus (crossed eyes) is a problem easily recognized and should receive immediate attention from a specialist. More subtle problems such as muscle imbalances, far-sightedness, and astigmatism are less easily detected and may not interfere noticeably with visual functioning until the child begins close work in school. Although use of vision for a variety of purposes may be one means of recognizing minor visual limitations, it is not necessarily the most critical. Cellular changes in general growth patterns may alter visual functioning. The eyeball and its internal structures continue to grow in size and shape until the teen years; this growth process alters the refractive components as well as the accommodative mechanisms so that a child may experience visual problems for the first time in the elementary or junior high years.

Without well-planned and regularly conducted visual screening programs during the school years, many children and youth with limited vision are never identified. The tragedy is that they may be labelled as academic failures, "dummies," or even mentally retarded—for no reason other than that their learning and achievement have been limited because no one has considered the possibility that they may have an undetected visual problem.

A carefully planned visual screening program should be conducted by trained personnel under the supervision of specialists in every community and should be a requirement in every school program. Screening is begun ideally in preschool years and repeated at regular intervals of every two or three years until at least the ninth grade. No child should be identified as learning disabled or mentally retarded without first having had a thorough visual examination and a battery of psychological tests.

After an identified visual problem has been referred to a specialist for diagnosis, some problems may be corrected by prescriptions for glasses or by a series of visual training exercises. A few children may require additional assistance in visual activities, and many can profit through the provision of special materials and equipment, at least until they reach maximum visual learning potential.

Organizational plans in public schools.   A survey of local school programs (Jones and Collins, 1966) showed five basic types of organizational patterns, ranging from the full-time, self-contained special class to the itinerant program in which a teacher-consultant serves children on a periodic basis but primarily provides materials and consultation to the regular classroom teacher. The question should be not which plan is best for any school district but instead, through which programming patterns can the children in that particular program be served most effectively.

Totally blind or very low-vision children whose developmental levels have not reached that of their sighted counterparts may require full-time special class placement with a specially trained teacher, at least until their learning and communication skills are developed to the point where they can participate fully with their sighted classmates in a regular program. Because totally blind children must use different materials and media for the basic learning-to-read and learning-to-write experiences, teachers for these children require specialized training.

For a long time, the general policy in local schools and in a few residential schools was to separate blind children from those who were called "partially seeing" for instructional purposes. This practice was probably a holdover from the period when very few teacher education programs were available, and those that existed had separate training programs for teachers of the blind and for teachers of the partially seeing. At present, teachers are educated as specialists to serve all visually handicapped children and youth. There is no longer any controversy about integrating in the same program blind children with those who have low vision or are visually limited, whether the delivery system is a special class, a resource room, or itinerant consultation (Jones and Collins, 1966).

Although no data on achievement of braille readers and print readers when instructed together have been reported in the United States, one study done in England (McLaughlin, 1974) recorded no noticeable difference in reading ability between braille readers and print readers in programs of integrated instruction. Logically, the similarity in learning ability is a more important factor than the nature or extent of the visual impairment. Children who find achievement difficult or who are not yet ready to develop such academic skills as reading, writing, and computation may need special class placement for a longer time. In fact, the current population of visually handicapped children, many of whom have other problems interfering with their development, has required local school districts to develop or reinstate self-contained and/or resource room programs to serve these children more effectively and to try to prevent the almost inevitable cumulative lag in educational development that occurs when the regular teacher tries to assume responsibilities for which she or he is not prepared.

In many local school settings, the majority of children at the elementary level are served through the *resource plan*. This plan involves selecting a particular school to which all visually handicapped children within that district are transported. This school contains a specially equipped classroom and a teacher trained to work with visually handicapped children. Children may be integrated into regular classes within that school for variable periods of time during the day or the week, according to the children's needs and the decisions of the special teacher and the regular teachers. Although this plan requires some children to be placed in settings other than their neighborhood schools, it does offer the children and the teacher a daily, sustained constellation of support services. In such a situation, some children who need more intensive assistance may spend several hours a day with the resource teacher in developing and refining social and academic skills (O'Brien, 1973); or, some children may spend the major portion of their time in the regular class with their peers, receiving only minimal assistance and consultative services from the resource teacher.

Itinerant services provide the opportunity for visually handicapped children to remain in their neighborhood schools and in regular classrooms with peers but still to be served by a specially qualified teacher on a periodic basis. Visually handicapped children then become the primary responsibility of the regular classroom teacher, with the consultative services of the special teacher and the provision of special equipment and materials adapted to their learning needs. For children and youths who have reached the level of being self-directive and independent in learning skills, these itinerant services would probably provide them with sufficient assistance; for children who have not yet developed their academic learning skills or who are not as socially developed as their sighted peers, this plan may offer less than the necessary range and intensive nature of the services actually needed by some children.

The number of children to be served on an intinerant basis should be determined by the characteristics of the individual children rather than by a specific number arrived at by a formula. This plan also requires a great deal of teacher time to be spent in travelling from school to school. The decision to establish such a procedure must be made on the basis of the effectiveness and efficiency of the plan for the children to be served, in addition to considering the appropriate use of time of a highly trained specialist.

Many school districts, especially large ones, and some of the smaller states in which there are strategic population centers find that a combination of resource and itinerant programs best meets the needs of their districts. Ideally, when visually handicapped children have reached the academic level of junior or senior high school, they have acquired sufficient independent learning and other skills so that they can progress consistently with minimal aid from itinerant special services. Many elementary-level visually handicapped children actually need the resource plan, and a few of the very young or slowly developing children will need self-contained situations for at least some time. Therefore, in large cities or heavily populated areas, probably the most effective pattern would be to provide early childhood education programs, self-contained classes, resource programs, and itinerant programs.

Of course, a total plan such as this is not feasible in areas where there are few visually handicapped children. The plan to utilize will have to be decided on the basis of the personnel available, the needs of the children in the program, and the numbers who require services. Conceivably, a local school district could use many or all of these patterns and vary them from year to year, according to the age and needs of the children to be served.

Residential programs.   States have traditionally established residential schools to provide educational experiences for severely visually handicapped children. A few smaller states have combined some of these programs with the programs for deaf children, and these have been known as "dual" schools. Formerly, all visually handicapped children within given states were sent to the residential school established specifically for them. However, as local schools began developing programs on a widespread basis, the approach to attendance in residential schools has varied from state to state and situation to situation.

There currently appears to be no overall policy followed by the greatest number of residential schools or states. In some cases, the residential school serves primarily children from remote, less populated areas of the state, those whose families for various reasons prefer to have them attend a residential program, or those children who simply cannot, for one reason or another, fit into the local school program in their community. In a few states, the residential school has ceased to serve children who can progress normally in academic learning, and all these children attend their local schools. Only those children who, because of the multiplicity of their problems, require a special curriculum different from that provided in the local schools are served by the state or private residential schools.

Many states are reevaluating their total special education programming for visually handicapped children in an effort to provide a range and continuum of educational services through a variety of organizational plans. For example, some states are planning to bring all programs and services together under one agency, thereby creating a continuum of services for the visually handicapped—from birth to vocational independence. The responsibility for coordinating such an agency would be one person's. In a few states, the traditional concept of the past 100 to 150 years has been maintained, meaning that there are virtually no programs in local public schools. So if visually handicapped children are to receive an education, they must attend the residential school. Still other states are expanding their residential programs to maintain the academic nature while providing a broader spectrum of programs for multihandicapped children in diagnostic services, daily living skills, and vocational programs. This expanded arrangement places an almost impossible task on the administration and is far more costly, to say nothing of the difficulties encountered in maintaining quality and diversity in the academic area.

In a few instances, the multihandicapped and vocational-skills programs are the main thrust of the school, although the schools continue to accept some students who are academically capable and pursue their education in the local community schools while they live at the residential school. No evidence is yet available to suggest the superiority of any one of these patterns or to indicate their effectiveness in accomplishing the objective of meeting their students' needs. Possibly within the next five to ten years, some national trends will lessen the present wide variability in local and residential school programs.

The following chart outlines a logical and feasible framework for a state-

State Plan for Services to Visually Handicapped Children and Youth

Program Levels and Living Arrangements	Disciplines and/or Personnel Involved	Nature and Scope of Services
	Physicians and eye specialists	Identification and reporting
Preschool and early childhood (0–9 years) Children live in own homes or foster homes	Public health nurses and social workers Preschool counselors and/or teachers Diagnostic and placement team	Case finding and referral Parental counseling and in-home teaching Local nurseries and kindergartens, programs in private agencies, preschool residential program, programs for multihandicapped
Elementary (6–14 years) Children live in own homes, foster homes, or regional residential centers	Physicians, therapists, and nurses Social workers and psychologists Special teachers, aides, mobility specialists, and counselors	Medical and therapeutic treatment Diagnostic and evaluation centers Local school programs, centers for multihandicapped, regional residential schools, screening and referral, parental counseling
Secondary (12–21 years) Youth live in own homes, foster homes, halfway houses, or regional residential settings	Vocational and/or career counselors, special teachers and aides, mobility specialists, psychologists and/or mental health counselors	Workshop training—sheltered workshops for multihandicapped; vocational or work-study on-the-job training Academic programs in local areas or regional residential center
Adult (18 years to independent, tax-paying citizens) Living arrangements with parents, in halfway houses, or independent setting	Vocational and/or career counselors Technical skills specialists Psychologists and/or mental health counselors Mobility specialists Placement specialists	Sheltered workshops Trade, technical, and/or vocational schools Business and professional schools Community colleges Senior colleges and/or universities

wide program that could serve as a guide-line for delivering comprehensive services. Personnel from numerous disciplines and community agencies would be employed at all stages; a variety of program services in several settings should be available; selection of service patterns and referrals to and from each program would be modified according to the needs and interests of the children, youth, and their parents at any stage. The potential for providing every necessary program and service within such a plan is unlimited. Coordination of a statewide plan would be challenging but the creative ideas that could be generated would help achieve the long-range goal of assuring independence early in the adult lives of visually handicapped youth.

Specialized Curriculum for the Visually Handicapped Child

The general practice in educational programming for visually handicapped children, especially in local schools, has been to parallel the academic curriculum of the sighted, although providing different materials, equipment, and teaching devices. The assumption that this enabled children to learn the same academic subjects that their sighted peers learned was not based on an objective appraisal of functional achievement. The tendency to parallel the regular school curriculum has been less prevalent in residential school programs. Although residential schools offered the same or similar academic subjects, they usually included many other subjects that were not considered appropriate for the visually handicapped in public schools—for example, physical education, homemaking, and shop. After federal legislation provided funds to establish teacher education programs across the entire field of special education, and with the expansion of educational research in teaching visually handicapped in colleges and universities and in the research division at the American Printing House for the Blind, mounting evidence began to indicate that greater attention should be given to selecting a specialized curriculum regardless of the location or type of program organization.

Some specialized aspects of the curriculum for visually handicapped students have been generally agreed on. In the sections that follow, we will discuss four broad areas and their specific emphases, in addition to some critical aspects of curriculum not often considered, and some of the variables affecting education of the visually handicapped.

1. Personal competencies and self-adjustment. This topic encompasses such activities of daily living as eating, dressing, and grooming skills; functional use of everyday materials and equipment in the home; social interactions with other people; sexual identity and preparation for marriage and family life; and homemaking and home management skills (Napier, 1973; Scholl, 1974; Suterko, 1973; Taylor, 1973). There seem to be two primary reasons for emphasizing such skills as part of the educational program. (1) Functional skills for living and adjustment are necessary for all persons, and since totally blind or very low-vision children and youth cannot acquire these skills incidentally by imitation of other people, teaching these skills should be a part of the educational program. (2) The child's self-concept and his feelings of social competence are dependent on his ability to demonstrate the same skills as his peers who have sight. The depth of this portion of the program must be determined by evaluating individual children's needs. In some cases, acquiring these functional skills may take precedence over academic learning experiences for a period of time. Social amenities of how to respond to other people and how to behave in certain social situations may be unknown to the child who is unable to monitor his environment or imitate the behavior of other people visually. Therefore, such social skills must be taught to children in settings where they can practice with understanding adults.

One facet of social and personal adjustment deserves special mention— that of sexual identity and preparation for marriage. Attitudes about self as a sexual being and an understanding of normal sexual development become relevant early in any child's life. These attitudes and understandings are formed according to whether, and in what way, questions arising out of the child's normal curiosity are answered or ignored. The nature of these attitudes emerges through the interplay of three factors: (1) the child's own impression of his sexual self, (2) the visual, audible, and tangible expressions of all those around the child, and (3) the child's own desire for sex education (Hooft and Heslinga, 1968). The normal learning through seeing a young baby bathed, viewing brothers and sisters in the nude, looking at pictures, and watching television and movies cannot be experienced by blind children, of course (Enis and Cataruzolo, 1972).

By the time visually handicapped youth reach high school and begin to think about relationships (and marriage) with those of the opposite sex, they may have many erroneous ideas or be totally ignorant of the basic facts relating to body parts and sexual functioning. Distorted ideas or lack of knowledge of consequences associated with sexual relationships could have tragic results. Courses in sex education and preparation for marriage and family life are absolutely necessary for visually handicapped children and youth. Suggestions and guidelines for planning such courses can be found in the references that follow (Kempton, 1975; Davidow, 1974; Dickman, 1972; Holmes, 1974; and the entire May issue of *The New Outlook for the Blind,* 1974).

2. Orientation, movement, and physical skills.   A second aspect of the specialized curriculum is teaching basic concepts related to orienting the body in relation to the environment and its contents, movement and travel within it, and acquiring skills related to recreational activities requiring physical agility. Chapter 3 presented a more thorough discussion of orientation and movement skills under the topic of psychomotor development. As students acquire basic knowledge of the body and its relationship to environmental space, mobility instructors can then teach them to move within that environ- ment without assistance. Students must be taught how to use a sighted guide for unfamiliar places, how to move independently by using a cane or a dog as a guide, and how to assess unfamiliar environments to anticipate appropri- ate movement patterns within them. Acquiring efficient travel skills requires long and intensive attention to physical activities and skills from a qualified mobility instructor.

Severely visually handicapped students may frequently be excluded from regular physical education activities, especially in public schools. Teachers may assume that they are incapable of participation or that they have no need to acquire certain physical skills. Physical education and recreational skills as a part of the school curriculum are probably more important for the health and fitness of visually handicapped students than for that of sighted students. Many of the physical activities and most of the competitive sports need to be modified or adapted for visually handicapped students to participate, but this participation provides a social interaction as well as a necessary positive image for the development of a strong self-concept. No adaptation is required for such activities as calisthenics, tumbling, or the standing broad jump. Minor adaptations are made in the rules of wrestling, requiring that contestants maintain body contact. Obviously, considerable adaptation must be made for blind students in competition running and in games requiring visual accuracy.

The importance of programming physical and recreational activities cannot be overemphasized because of their importance to the total life adjustment and functioning of visually handicapped individuals. Unfortunately, however, too little attention is given to them and numerous youth must go to rehabilitation centers for such training after they complete their schooling.

3. Communication skills.   The first component requiring special emphasis in the academic curriculum is communication. Communication skills refer to the special types of competencies needed in reading, listening, writing, and speaking. These skills bear a strong relation to affective and psychomotor development as well as to cognitive development. The more efficient the individual is in acquiring information, in responding to those in his world, and in functioning in all aspects of learning and living, the stronger will be his confidence in himself and his feelings that he is a capable human being.

Differences of opinion continue unsettled in relation to the development of reading skills in visually handicapped students. For those who are totally blind, the primary reading skill to be developed as soon as the child is ready to learn to read is obviously tactual reading. Even under the best circumstances, braille reading is a slower means of gathering information after the first few years of becoming familiar with the process; there is little difference in reading speed between braille reading as compared to print reading during the first two or three years of school life (Nolan and Kederis, 1969). However, after this time, even the best braille readers are unable to achieve the same speed in reading as the sighted reader. Part of the efficiency in braille reading is related to the knowledge and recognition of the symbols. Therefore, teachers should strongly emphasize training in recognizing the braille symbols as a means of increasing reading speed. (A more thorough discussion of braille follows later in this chapter.)

Deciding which medium to use for reading is more difficult with the low-vision child, since not all teachers agree on the criteria for selecting the appropriate approach to reading with such children. Jones (1961) found a wide variation in the reading medium (braille or print) in children having varying degrees of visual acuity. Some children with extremely low vision were found to be print readers, whereas other children with much higher visual acuity were found to be braille readers. Studies by Barraga (1964) and Ashcroft, Halliday, and Barraga (1966) have indicated that, when given an appropriate program in visual stimulation and visual perceptual development, low-vision children can be effective visual learners. This may be a long process for some children, depending on other individual characteristics such as motivation, intelligence, and readiness to learn visually. Teachers are sometimes eager to decide quickly which is the best reading medium and approach to use with children. As a consequence, because of the slow process of learning to read visually for some children, teachers assume that they would be better readers through the use of braille. However, observation and experience have indicated that if children have visual capabilities, they will attempt to use them.

There was a period of time when children were actually blindfolded or in some other way kept from looking at braille so that they would not learn to read with their eyes. This controversy has probably been settled by this time and the tenet generally accepted that if a child can see to read braille with his eyes, then for goodness' sake, give him something easier to read with the eyes than braille! Children who have limited visual functioning and whose visual reading is slow and requires specific materials and optimal lighting conditions may need to learn to read in both braille and print. Whether or not confusion results from the concurrent learning of print and braille symbols has not yet been determined. However, many think that children could learn to read using braille and print simultaneously; classroom experiments using this approach have been quite effective with selected children. The decision appears to rest with the individual child, his learning capacities, and his coding and processing abilities. Whatever the medium selected, helping the child achieve the highest possible efficiency should be one of the primary objectives of any specialized program.

Information can also be gathered through the auditory sense. For this reason, acquiring listening skills is an important aspect of learning for visually handicapped students. Several teachers and teacher educators have developed programs for teaching listening skills (Bishop, 1971; Simpkins, 1971; Tait, 1973). Teaching listening skills should begin in the early educational years and receive increased emphasis as visually handicapped students progress through their school years. Even though junior and senior high school students will probably (and should) continue to use either braille or print reading for much of their school learning, efficiency in acquiring information suggests that they should begin to rely more on listening as a primary source of information.

Nolan (1966) compared braille reading with listening and found that listening to recorded material required only about one-third the time required for tactual reading of the same material and that no loss in comprehension was experienced. Several studies relating to using accelerated speech for listening have indicated that there is no difference in comprehension between material presented at a normal rate of speech, that presented at a compressed rate, and the same material presented in braille. Studies do show, however, that "reading" by listening to compressed speech was more efficient from the standpoint of both speed and comprehension than either reading through braille or reading by listening to a recording at a normal rate of speech.

The nature of the material seemed to have some relationship to the comprehension through listening, whether the material was presented at a normal rate or at an accelerated rate (Gore, 1969; Tuttle, 1972). Comprehension of scientific and other abstract material decreased as the rate of presentation increased. Foulke (1969) has presented some negative aspects of reading by listening. For example, without special devices for slowing or accelerating the rate of taped material, the listener has little control over the rate at which he is able to "read"; there is difficulty in listening ahead or in going back over material already heard; and fewer contextual clues are available through listening than from either braille or print. Despite the lack of detailed knowledge regarding efficiency, specialists agree generally that skill in listening for the purpose of "reading" is an important part of the educational program for all visually handicapped students.

Writing skills are another aspect of communication that require particular emphasis. For totally blind children, using the braille writer for beginning writing skills is usually incorporated with braille reading, so that children acquire both reading and writing simultaneously. Transfer to the use of the more portable slate and stylus is recommended by the later elementary years, since junior and senior high school students will find this method more efficient for taking notes and for their own purposes. Some of the advantages of the braille writer for younger children are that less fine motor coordination is required to use the writer, and what the child has written is available immediately in an upright position for scanning or checking. In contrast, paper must be turned over and the slate removed to read what is written by stylus, since the dots are depressed. (Using the slate and stylus requires the mental ability to reverse the position of dot numbers in the braille cell.) Writing with the slate and stylus is done from left to right since the braille dots are punched down instead of up, as is the case with the braille writer. Developing efficiency in braille writing is a necessity for all totally blind students so that they will be able to communicate among themselves and also monitor sentence structure for academic work.

There is disagreement about the proper stage in the elementary program at which to introduce typing to totally blind and very low-vision students. As soon as the child has acquired competent braille writing skills (probably about the third or fourth grade), he is usually able to learn to type many of his lessons. Teaching him the touch-typing method is the responsibility of the specially trained teacher and should be a part of his curriculum. In some residential schools, typing may not be introduced until the sixth grade or even as late as the eighth grade in some schools. The child's need to communicate with his regular class teacher in the local school or with his family (if he attends a residential school) often dictates the time at which the child is taught typing; his own interest and ability are other factors to consider.

Introducing typing as early as seems appropriate for the individual may be valuable for strengthening spelling skills and perhaps also for fostering mental memory, since the visually handicapped typist must remember not only what he has typed but also what is to follow in order to be aware of location within the paragraph and on the page. Since visual monitoring is impossible in many instances, developing accuracy is of great importance. As soon as the child in public school is able to become efficient in typing, he can prepare his own work. This ability may influence the extent to which he can be integrated with his sighted peers and achieve success in the regular classroom.

The process and technique of teaching low-vision children or visually limited children how to write is different from that used with normally seeing children. Rather than teaching manuscript letters to low-vision children and and most visually limited children, it is more appropriate to teach cursive writing from the very beginning. These children have great difficulty developing skill in manuscript writing since the pencil or pen must be relocated each time a letter is formed. In addition, spacing is difficult to judge when vision is poor, so learning from the start to connect the letters in cursive writing is easier and more logical. However, learning to form the letters and to join them will take a longer period of time than with normally sighted children and will require more assistance. Legibility rather than perfection is the primary goal.

Totally blind children also should be taught to use the same writing materials as seeing children and learn at least to write their own names. Previously, we have tended to wait until just before a student graduated from school to teach him to write his name. Because he had little concept of the nature of print symbols, much less of how to form them, learning to write his name was a difficult task for the student, and for many youth virtually impossible. The trend now is to emphasize handwriting early for totally blind children, probably when they begin to show interest in their own names and want to use pencils just as other people do.

Some teachers advocate teaching handwriting along with braille writing to permit children to become acquainted with both braille symbols and print symbols as a means of facilitating the association between them. From the standpoint of psychomotor development, it would be appropriate to teach blind children to write at the chalkboard first, since gross movements would be easier than the finer movements required by pencil and paper. Then, once they had learned letter formations, writing might be transferred to sheets of aluminum foil, so that they could feel what they had written. Some materials are designed specifically to produce raised lines that are discriminable tactually. Some blind children learn to write script well and can thereby communicate with their sighted classmates to some extent.

Developing spoken communication is especially relevant for effective interpersonal and vocational interactions as well as for conferences or committee work. Because visually handicapped students are unable to see the speaker or audience to read their nonverbal cues, such things as eye contact, facing the speaker or audience, voice projection, and coherent, organized expression of thought should be developed through planned strategies. A course in spoken communications for junior or senior high school students could be designed to include some of the following topics, similar to those suggested by Simon (1974): (1) interviewing, (2) conversation, (3) small-group communication, (4) listening and receiving information and responding, (5) appropriate language and coherent expression, and (6) nonverbal communication. For older students, planning, organizing, and presenting a public speech for communicating an idea is a useful project.

Applying this discussion to the children depicted in the first section, Carl would very probably be able to learn to write his name during his early school years; Lucy should certainly be taught to write simultaneously with learning to read, and she would probably be able to develop a legible script. Dora and Keith, who would have already known how to write before they lost their vision, should be encouraged to continue writing, since if they did not, they would be likely to lose this motor skill.

There is a close interrelationship between these aspects of the specialized curriculum and the overall academic and personal-social achievement of visually handicapped students. How they feel about themselves is related to the number and variety of skills they are able to acquire, and which approximate those of their sighted peers.

4. Prevocational information.   The fourth dimension of the special curriculum is introducing the types of vocations and careers possible and the skills required for each. What people do, how they do it, and what is required of an individual to perform a certain job is information not commonly available to the visually handicapped student. Therefore, communicating the understanding that arithmetic, spelling, and other subject matter are related to, or may prepare him for, a future vocation should be considered an important part of the total educational curriculum. Chapter 9 is devoted to a discussion of this subject.

Educational Media

Providing educational materials for visually handicapped students comparable to the wide variety of materials available for normally seeing students has posed problems throughout the years, and many of these have yet to be solved. The educational "materials explosion" has motivated increased research into learning in the visually handicapped and has created an impetus for greater experimentation and adaptation of media and materials. Those materials and devices specifically designed for the use of visually handicapped students are discussed in this section.

Braille codes.   After years of controversy, the basic braille cell of six dots designed by Louis Braille has now been accepted internationally as the one graphic symbol for use by blind readers. The sixty-three possible dot combinations form the basis for the literary braille code, a music code, a mathematical code, and a scientific code. The variety of codes developed from this basic six-dot braille cell and all possible combinations thereof has been likened to a series of foreign languages. The multiple arrangements of symbols, the use of the same symbols to have a variety of meanings depending on their relation to other symbols or because of their particular spatial position, and the many arbitrary rules for using these symbols make all braille codes complex language systems for interpretation. A sophisticated system of braille shorthand in the form of contractions, letter combinations, and shortened forms of words saves space and usually time in reading; however, such extensive abbreviation may increase the time required for interpretation and recognition of new words in unfamiliar contexts, although it increases efficiency in reading more familiar material (Henderson, 1973; Lowenfeld, 1973; Nolan and Kederis, 1969). In braille codes, it is impossible to maintain the sound-symbol relationship found in print symbols; this sound-symbol inconstancy poses an additional difficulty in recognition.

Directly translating printed books used in the early school years into braille presents a serious problem because of the difficulty of recognition. Words easily recognized by sight may be difficult when transcribed into braille. The difficulty level of reading material for children in the first few years of school may suggest designing "controlling symbols," or special reading materials specifically for those children who will use braille (Rex, 1970), in order to introduce gradually the difficult word symbols of the braille literary code. Long-term research projects should be designed and conducted to evaluate the efficiency of various braille literary code abbreviations in facilitating learning to read.

Regardless of the process of learning or the methodologies used, the braille-reading child will be required throughout his school years to refine his skills of recognition and his knowledge of the various aspects of the code and its multiple uses. Those young people who intend to continue in academic and literary pursuits beyond high school will find even greater challenges in the use of Grade 3 braille, an even more abbreviated, but more efficient and space-saving, form for adult use.

The Optacon.   The development of the Optacon by Linville and Bliss (1965) and the eventual refinement of this optical-to-tactile conversion instrument, now manufactured by Telesensory Systems, has generated considerable interest among educators and rehabilitation personnel. As a transistorized "retina" built into a tiny camera passes over print symbols, the image is converted to a tactual representation of the letter shape, which is then perceived on the forefinger of the blind person. This requires that the blind person know the shape of print letters and be able to recognize them tactually. Whether or not this is a feasible reading method for totally blind children is not yet known, although one project (the San Diego Project, 1971) suggests that some young children may be able to use the Optacon to read regular print material as early as the first or second grade.

Other studies (Bliss and Moore, 1974; Moore, 1973) indicate that a number of variables are primary determinants in the effectiveness of the Optacon as a reading device. These studies indicate that a high level of intellectual functioning is one critical consideration, along with long periods of training and consistent use, plus the motivation of the reader to spend the time and energy necessary to gain efficiency using this device. At best, reading rates are slow and have yet to surpass the reading rate in braille for these same individuals. However, the fact that print material may be read without modification or transcription makes the Optacon worthy of further study. Some studies now in progress with school-age children may reveal this to be a valuable technological invention. At present, the cost of the instrument is prohibitive for widespread use in the schools or privately.

Large print and magnification.   A visual image may be enlarged in three ways: (1) increasing the size of the material itself (large print), (2) bringing the image or material closer to the eye, or (3) using a device to magnify the size of the material. The accepted notion for a number of years was that large-print materials would be easier to see for the visually limited and low-vision child. Studies reported inconclusive and often contradictory evidence regarding the size of type most easily read (Eakin, Pratt, and McFarland, 1961; Nolan, 1959). Further studies relating to school achievement and the effect of type size on reading and achievement (Bateman and Weatherall, 1967; Birch, Tisdall, Peabody, and Sterrett, 1966) suggest that type size has little to do with reading speed or comprehension in visually limited children.

Two ophthalmologists, Faye (1970) and Fonda (1966), have said that many children may have been encouraged or even forced to read large-print books and materials when, in fact, they could more easily have read material in regular print size, either with or without magnification. Sykes (1971, 1972) found that high school students, when provided with magnifying devices from which to choose and special lamps and/or lighting arrangements, were just as efficient with regular sized print materials as they were with large-print materials; in fact, some with lower degrees of measured vision were even more efficient with regular sized type. Reading standard print was found to be no more tiring than reading large print, implying that the concern should be not with the size of the type but with the quality of the print and the illumination. There may be a few children who are able to function visually only when they have large type and perhaps even magnification. In such cases, using large-print materials may be indicated, depending on individual children and their motivation to function visually.

Producing large-type textbooks is expensive, and the pictures in these textbooks are often more difficult for visually limited children to use than the color pictures in regular textbooks would be. Because of the expense, the number of titles available in large print is limited (Goldish, 1968). Most of these textbooks are very large and too bulky for children to handle easily; in addition, they look so different from standard books that some children are embarrassed to use them.

The refinement in quality of nonprescription magnifiers and the development of low-vision aid clinics that prescribe aids individually for children who are unable to use regular refractive lenses (or for whom lenses to be worn on the face are inappropriate) has resulted in a trend toward increased use of magnifying devices. Neither visual acuity measurements nor the nature of the visual defect seems to have any relationship to the children's ability to use either large-print materials or magnification devices or low-vision aids. Experiments with closed-circuit television as a means of enlarging reading material indicate that this may be a promising method for future use. Again, however, the prohibitive cost of such systems will probably delay widespread use for many years.

When children cannot be fitted with optical aids that enable them to function with some visual efficiency, using hand-held or stand magnifiers is the most feasible solution. There is still worldwide controversy regarding large print and visual aids. It is doubtless more logical to consider *both* as possible ways for children to function more efficiently visually rather than to take an either-or position. The decision should really be made in relation to the individual child, his visual condition, and his motivation to function with either large type or magnification. There is some indication that as reading efficiency increases in children, they may be able to transfer from the use of large type or magnification to regular sized materials and still maintain equal speed and comprehension.

The style, spacing, and density of print are significant variables to consider. Teachers should be careful to provide many different print sizes, styles, and so forth to enable children to choose what is best for them. Because the letters appear to run together, large, bold type with letters spaced close together is more difficult to read than smaller type with letters spaced farther apart. Letters with less density are difficult to discriminate. The most visible print is simple in style, moderately bold, and well spaced. Lighting is also a critical factor; some children need more light or light directed onto the material, whereas others can function more efficiently with less direct or intense light. Again, teachers should let the child try many different lighting conditions to permit him to select the optimal condition for him.

All optical aids and some magnifiers require a long period of time and much patience and training before children can use them effectively. Proper use of optical aids and magnifiers cannot be left to chance. If training is not available through the clinic or specialist that provides the aid, then the teacher must give whatever special training the child needs—otherwise the aid will be rejected and learning may be unnecessarily inhibited.

Rather than continuing to engage in argument in an attempt to establish the superiority of one type of material or one means of enlarging reading material over another, a more reasonable approach is to try all materials and devices that might facilitate a higher level of visual functioning in all visually handicapped children. Lighting conditions, especially the use of individual tensor lights, and seating arrangements in the classroom according to the child's preferences require careful attention. In addition, greater use of rear-view projection devices, individual, desk-sized projectors, and overhead projection machines (provided that the projected image is large, the contrast is sharp, and that the children can choose the distance and angle of viewing) should be encouraged.

Abacus and computational devices.   The search for an effective device for blind students to make arithmetic computations resulted in the development of a variety of gadgets and computational aids, none of which has enabled the blind student to function in computational skills comparable to sighted students. Many programs began to use the Perkins Brailler to simulate the same format in setting up problems as that used by sighted students with pencil and paper. Computation, however, is an abstract mental activity, and difficulties continued. Eventually the Numberaid, Calculaid, and an adaptation of the Japanese abacus, designed by Cranmer, were made available by the American Printing House for the Blind. A recent study (Lewis, 1970) found that sixty-six percent of the school programs were using the Cranmer abacus, although some were continuing to use the braille writer. The abacus was ranked as being of greatest value to blind students for computation. Nevertheless, Brothers (1972) found that arithmetic computation continued to be a critical concern among educators. According to Brothers, there seem to be several possible alternatives: "(1) the use of the Numberaid or other concrete manipulative device at the third and fourth grade level, (2) providing an opportunity for all students to become proficient with the abacus by the completion of grade six, and (3) placing much less emphasis on the braille writer as a computational aid" (p. 7).

Although the problems in computation for blind students have not yet been resolved, it is clear that easy-to-handle computational aids should be made available during the child's early school life for arithmetic concepts to be thoroughly understood. These devices may also be useful for students with low vision—for example, supplementing pencil-and-paper computational skills with the Numberaid and abacus to increase efficiency. No single process or device has been identified as the most appropriate for all children. Thus, teachers should continue to experiment with various approaches to permit severely visually handicapped students to acquire computational skills and to achieve in arithmetic at a level comparable to that of their sighted peers.

Other media and equipment.   Concrete objects and materials known as "realia," which may be purchased commercially or gathered from general environmental sources, are valuable for teaching basic concepts and should be a part of every classroom during the early educational years. Models and miniature three-dimensional representations of objects appear to have little use in the first few grades, because the great discrepancy in size and texture between the model and reality may be confusing to visually handicapped children until concepts of real objects are well established. As the students grow older and are able to make the association and transfer through abstract thinking, models may come to have some use, especially for representing large or inaccessible objects (Napier, 1973). Although the value of three-dimensional models and two-dimensional representations was studied a number of years ago, little recent attention has been given to determining the relative usefulness or inappropriateness of such materials.

The use of talking-book machines and records made especially for visually handicapped students for recreational reading is well known. The development of cassette tape recorders has permitted greater use of such equipment for many more children because of the portability and the fact that each student may employ this equipment for his personal needs, wherever he may be and in whatever educational setting he studies. Record players, tape recorders, audio-card readers, and cassette playback machines should be integral to every program for visually handicapped children. With such equipment, teachers may prepare individual instructions for independent work, and students may even tape their responses. These machines help to replace the chalkboard and are time-savers for both students and teachers. The relative benefits of using prepared programmed instructional materials have not yet been sufficiently explored. Continued interest of engineers and other specialists in developing mechanical and electronic devices for instructing blind persons will ensure further refinement of materials and devices to enhance the learning and the functioning of severely visually handicapped students.

8   Assessment and Evaluation of Individual Functioning

Throughout the field of education, the question of assessment and evaluation is still a worrisome matter because of the questionable validity of some tests and the unreliability of the scores obtained. This fact is especially true in special education when considering using psychological and educational evaluation of present functioning in visually handicapped children for possible predictive purposes. Since many educators working with visually handicapped children are not psychologists, and since many psychologists have had little opportunity to study the effects of reduced vision or total lack of vision on children's behavioral responses, communication between the fields and coordinated approaches to evaluating individual functioning are even more difficult to come by.

For a period of time, there seemed to be a need to test and assess visually handicapped children both psychologically and educationally to compare their development and functioning with that of sighted children, but using measurement scales and test instruments designed for, and standardized primarily on, sighted children. In gathering such information and reporting the results, very little distinction was made between children who were totally blind and those who had usable vision. Obviously, the use of contaminated samples called into question the validity of the findings and negated the possibility of generalizing to a total population with only one characteristic in common—visual impairment.

Despite the fact that visually handicapped children and youth as a group were found to function psychologically and educationally at levels below those of sighted children of the same age, more complete evidence has shown that in reality many children seemed to achieve just as well or better in academic work and were able to perform at comparable levels or above in real-life situations. Contradictory observations of this nature have caused both psychologists and educators to examine not only the procedures used in evaluation but also to call into question the entire approach toward assessment and evaluation as applied to visually handicapped children.

Critical issues and questions raised by Bateman (1965), Weiner (1967), and Chase (1972) indicate that more careful examination should be given to a wide variety of variables and approaches. Prior to any testing or assessment, the following questions should be considered.

1. For what purpose is the assessment being made? Is it to exclude the child from some program or service, or is it to prove that he is eligible to be included? Is assessment for the purpose of prediction, or is it an attempt to determine present level of functioning? Is the primary purpose to demonstrate the need for a more realistic learning program? Is evaluation done to provide a base from which to assess the child's progress in learning in relation to his own performance, or is it to make a comparison with other blind children or with sighted children of comparable age?
2. Are definitive norms or age-level equivalents required or desirable? If so, should assessment tools and measures designed for sighted children be utilized, or should specific measures and tools be designed for blind children?
3. Are the criteria used in the assessment process related to what is desired or to what one is likely to find? Can the same criteria be applied to totally blind children that are applied to low-vision children? If not, how should these criteria differ?
4. In evaluating functioning, how does one determine whether a lower level of functioning (either below or above that anticipated) is due to lack of experience or opportunity to learn, or whether the child is incapable of learning? On the other hand, is the higher level of functioning due to an enriched background of experience, or does the child simply have greater learning capacity and has he learned in spite of lack of opportunity?
5. How does the person doing the assessment determine whether an inappropriate response or behavior is due to the visual problem or the fact that the child may have a neurological or learning problem?

Substantial information about whether tactual and auditory experiences are analogous to visual experiences is lacking. Possible differences in how various sensory systems process the data received could influence learning styles and patterns. But to this time, these differences in information processing have eluded assessment through present instruments and procedures. Despite these perplexing questions, assessing functional behavior can be valuable to the child, to the teachers attempting to work with the child, and to the parents. Thus, instead of rejecting the idea of evaluating visually handicapped children because we do not agree about how to go about the process, a better approach would seem to be to suggest how the procedure could be improved and which measures and procedures are most valuable to individual children.

Range and Type of Behavior
to Be Evaluated

Intelligence.   Hayes (1952) attempted to adapt the Binet materials into an instrument known as the Interim Hayes-Binet to assess the mental ability of visually handicapped children. The work was never completed, although the cut-and-paste version served well for a number of years. Validity at some age levels and overall reliability were left in doubt. However, individual measures of mental development and learning abilities (usually referred to as "intelligence tests") may be appropriate evaluative tools when used by sensitive, qualified psychologists who are cautious and fair in their interpretation of the information received.

The verbal portion of the Wechsler Intelligence Scales is probably the most widely used single measure. Some studies have shown a positive correlation between scores on these verbal measures and future academic success in school. However, Tillman (1967) found that there were many things visually handicapped children had simply not had the opportunity to learn and were therefore unable to provide a standard reply. The performance on vocabulary items showed the lack of knowledge about things, but perhaps the most noticeable effect of the lack of visual learning and processing was the inability to give similarities between things. By the age of sixteen, at which time the Wechsler Adult Intelligence Scale (WAIS) was used, many of these discrepancies in responses had disappeared. Even at this time, though, there were differences between the responses of blind and sighted youth of the same age.

A long-time concern has been to develop a means of evaluating functional intelligence as a possible predictive basis for learning potential on performance tasks. Efforts through the years (Dauterman, Shapiro, and Suinn, 1967) have failed to produce a performance scale for the visually handicapped that might be comparable to those on standard intellectual measures for children and youth under sixteen years of age. The long-term nature of such projects, the great expense, and the difficulty in finding sufficient numbers for standardization samples have been some of the problems related to these endeavors.

One measure of functional intelligence, Bauman's Nonlanguage Learning Test (1973), is primarily a clinical instrument that employs formboards. It is adaptable for use with many age groups since the nature of the tasks can be varied according to the performance of the individual. The formboard consists of eight holes of various shapes into which can be inserted two, three, or four pieces to form the required shape. Bauman suggests that interpretation is facilitated by carefully observing the reaction of the child or person being assessed. Furthermore, interpretation of performance becomes more valid with continued trials. No standardization has been attempted.

The Blind Learning Aptitude Test (BLAT), based on abstract symbol discrimination, recognition, and association, uses culturally neutral items designed to sample certain psychological processes considered important in the act of learning (Newland, 1961). Memory and verbal adequacy are not required. Test items are presented in bas-relief on heavy plastic, and except where textural contrast is necessary, the items are constructed of embossed dots. Total configurations are larger than the traditional braille cell. Minimal emphasis is placed on what the child has learned previously so that the predictive potential for future learning is uncontaminated.

Two performance measures that have some standardization norms for use above the age of sixteen are the Haptic Intelligence Scale (HIS) (Surrager and Surrager, 1964) and the Stanford-Kohs Block Design Test (Suinn and Dauterman, 1966). The HIS has six subtests designed to supplement the WAIS verbal scale and intended to assess certain mental functioning not evaluated through verbal responses. One study (Streitfeld and Avery, 1968) found a strong correlation between the HIS and the verbal portion of the WAIS and concluded that the information from the HIS added little to the prediction of achievement that was not obtained through the WAIS verbal scale.

Little evidence has been gathered regarding the validity or predictive value of the Stanford-Kohs Block Design Test. The single task is to arrange the blocks into various patterns of increasing complexity according to tactually perceived designs. The standardization sample was small, and no norms are available below sixteen years of age. However, there does seem to be some possible value in using this assessment measure to determine how a student approaches a task and to estimate problem-solving ability. Perhaps some studies would clarify the validity and reliability of this measure.

More recently, the 1960 Stanford-Binet has been adapted in two forms— Form N for subjects with no usable vision, and Form U for those with usable vision—and has been standardized on sighted, blind, and visually limited children. This measure is known as the Perkins-Binet (Davis, 1970). Availability for widespread use is expected in the near future. The fact that thirty percent of the items in Form N and twenty-five percent of those in Form U are performance items may help minimize the overemphasis on assessment of verbal abilities, since only the verbal section of the WISC is used as a predictor of intellectual potential and functioning (Coveny, 1972).

These various measures of intellectual assessment may provide valuable clinical data and some pertinent information for educational planning; however, great caution should be exercised in their interpretation since there is no evidence yet to establish the validity of intelligence test scores as reliable indicators of learning potential or academic achievement in visually handicapped children.

Nevertheless, teachers would like to use information from psychological reports of intellectual assessment to help them plan realistically for children. They want to know children's strengths and weaknesses in specific learning areas and may be unable to make such inferences from scores on tests or subtests. Psychometrists and psychologists would provide a real service to teachers and children if they would specify the mental processes evaluated in certain tasks and indicate the areas of intellectual deficits.

In addition to, or instead of, using single measures to obtain IQ scores, selected subtests from several measures could provide useful information for educational planning. Bullard and Barraga (1971) analyzed the subtests of numerous evaluative instruments and organized them according to the type of mental task required in each. The following categories were identified: (1) immediate recall, (2) association, (3) logical thinking, (4) discrimination, (5) spatial relations, (6) deductive reasoning, (7) inductive reasoning, (8) imitation, (9) generalization, (10) attention span, and (11) language development. Sampling intellectual functions in such a manner would not yield scores but could result in a profile of functional abilities and deficits useful for prescriptive planning of learning experiences.

Social maturity. The Maxfield-Buchholz Scale (1957) of social maturity, adapted from the Vineland and standardized on preschool blind children, is used to test personal, social, and functional development in handicapped children. Covering a variety of physical, social, and self-directive dimensions of development, the first items are related primarily to physical control of the body, eating, dressing, and finally to communication and self-direction at the four-, five- and six-year levels. Although this scale was designed to be administered through interview with the parents, usage through the years has indicated that a valid assessment of developmental skills could also be obtained through personal observation in actual settings, supplemented by parental, teacher, and houseparent interviews. In addition to evaluating social maturity, the teacher can infer many aspects of mental functioning from this scale. Items from some of the preschool measures have been recognized as useful indexes of several aspects of mental growth.

Achievement. Achievement testing of visually handicapped students has occurred since the early 1900s. The American Printing House for the Blind has published a variety of achievement tests in braille, and in 1967, the first large-type achievement test was published. More recently, the 1973 Stanford Achievement Test series has been adapted for use with visually handicapped students (Morris, 1974). All levels, except Primary Level I (which has been omitted because of its extensive pictorial content), for grades 1.5 to 2.4 have been modified and are available in braille and in large type. According to Morris (1974, p. 39), "The Stanford Achievement Test series holds promise of being the most useful to date." This series is important because it will be possible to rank visually handicapped students in relation to their sighted counterparts. Further use of the achievement tests may provide the opportunity for local school programs and residential schools to develop norms specifically for visually handicapped students in addition to comparing their progress with their sighted peers'.

The earlier practice in many schools of having the special teacher read the achievement test to the student and mark his responses for him invalidates the procedures as well as the validity of the scores obtained. Now that all levels of the Stanford Achievement Test are available in braille and large type, with appropriate time adjustments, there is no reason not to give achievement tests to all visually handicapped students.

The Scholastic Aptitude Test (SAT) and other aptitude measures are also available in both braille and large type, for those who wish to pursue their education beyond high school. Waiving the SAT or the Graduate Record Examination (GRE) for blind students, a practice followed in many colleges and universities, has no basis now and could be detrimental to some students.

Special skills. Evaluating the efficiency with which visually handicapped children use their sensory abilities is valuable in planning individualized programs, especially in relation to the tactual sense and the use of residual vision. The Roughness Discrimination Test (RDT) was designed as a tool to measure the development of the ability to make coordinated tactual discriminations with the hands and fingers, which, of course, is important for learning to read braille (Nolan and Morris, 1965). The measure was validated with groups of first-grade children, showing that children who do well on the RDT at the beginning of the first grade tend to be successful in learning to read braille; those who did poorly were less likely to be successful (Nolan and Morris, 1965). The American Printing House for the Blind has made available tactual discrimination worksheets, which may be used to assess skill in discriminating geometric forms, lines, angles, and braille characters—all of which are indicators of readiness to perceive and understand braille symbols. The RDT and the worksheets not only accurately assess young children's tactual discrimination ability, but they are also designed to be administered by teachers in the classroom. The advantage is that no special training is required for administration and no clinical interpretation is necessary.

The Visual Efficiency Scale (Barraga, 1970) was designed to assess the level of visual functioning through a series of increasingly smaller and less visible items, sequenced in complexity from gross form to visual detail to words and sentences. The primary purpose of this measure is to determine the degree of visual efficiency with which children are able to function even though they have visual impairments. The scale was planned primarily for use with low-vision students, who might previously have been considered unable to use their residual vision for learning purposes. The scale may also be useful for those with less severe visual problems who have difficulty discriminating specific types of detailed materials or whose difficulties are related to perceptual problems. The VES (Visual Efficiency Scale) and the *Teacher's Guide for Development of Visual Learning Abilities and Utilization of Low Vision* (Barraga, 1970) have received both national and international acceptance, having been translated into several foreign languages.

A profile of visual efficiency is drawn from performance, which indicates a low level, a marginal level, or a satisfactory level of visual functioning. The validity and reliability for preschool sighted children and low-vision children from six to fourteen years of age have been established (Harley, Spollen, and Long, 1973; Harley and Spollen, 1973). Content validity and internal consistency among items were established with both groups. Definitive research to establish the relationship between the visual performance on this scale and subsequent visual learning has not yet been completed. No predictions of potential learning abilities or efficiency can be made from the functional assessment acquired from the VES. A decided advantage is that the scale can be administered by teachers and used as a guide for planning visual experiences and activities.

Other special-skills assessment measures and tools are available, although many of them lack specific standardization or reliability criteria. Some of these are the Anxiety Scale for the Blind (Hardy, 1968), the Adolescent Emotional Factors Inventory (Bauman, 1963), and a number of manual dexterity measures. Most of these are open to clinical interpretation and may not be suitable for use by other than trained psychologists. Only a few of these are appropriate for use with school-age children and youth. The Minnesota Rate of Manipulation, the Penn Bi-Manual Work Sample, and the Crawford Small Parts Dexterity Test are all measures to assess the speed and efficiency of manipulation with tools and materials.

Special Considerations in Evaluation and Assessment

For whatever purpose the child is being assessed or whoever the person (whether a psychologist or a teacher) doing the evaluation, several critical variables determine whether the evaluation provides meaningful information. If the child is totally blind, then it is important to know whether that child has been blind from birth (as in the case of Carl) or whether the child lost vision through either a deteriorating condition or an accident (such as in the cases of Dora and Keith). If loss of vision occurred after the child had learned to function visually, the age of onset of blindness is another important variable. For totally blind students to feel at ease and for them to understand the nature of the task and what the evaluator expects them to do requires a special method of presentation. Standard instructions used with sighted persons are often inappropriate and confusing, leaving the child wondering what he is to do and how he is to do it. Instructions should be clear and concise, permitting only one interpretation of the task to be performed. If the test is to be timed, the child should be told this so that he clearly understands that he is to work with the greatest possible speed and efficiency.

The information gathered from children who have usable vision performing a task that is primarily tactual may be less easily interpreted, since it is difficult to know to what degree their remaining vision has enhanced the performance. An effective procedure might be to blindfold such students in order to obtain valid results. In contrast, when the task is primarily visual and the person has very limited visual capability, it is difficult to determine whether the inability to perform a task is related to the visual impairment or whether the task has not been understood. It is especially difficult for low-vision children to perform visual tasks with speed—a factor that needs to be taken into consideration. This is another difficulty related to using evaluative materials designed for sighted individuals, especially when the performance of those who are visually limited will be compared with the performance of those who are normally seeing. Although the visually limited child is perfectly capable of performing the same task, he is likely to require more time.

Comprehensive Assessment Plan for Use in Educational Settings

Any extensive plan of behavioral evaluation includes information from a multitude of disciplines, representative samples of behavior in numerous situations, and both observational and objective data from parents, social workers, teachers, psychologists, and medical specialists. The objective of evaluation at any age should be to make practical judgments and decisions regarding appropriate interventions to increase performance and determine the effectiveness or ineffectiveness of previously used strategies.

An overall plan for organizing and selecting the assessment to be made enhances the usefulness of the evaluative information obtained. Weiner (1967) suggested a framework within which to consider behavioral responses. The *level of performance* indicates how much development has taken place in any dimension and the point from which to design future learning tasks. The length of time required to achieve a certain stage of development or learning is indicative of the *rate* at which gains may be expected. The *range* of behavior suggests the array of learning opportunities provided for functioning in a broad spectrum of activities. Accuracy or behavioral adequacy in relation to speed of performance characterizes the *efficiency* of achievement to be anticipated. *Autonomous behavior* is perceived as independence when self-initiated and self-directed tasks are approached and executed without instruction; approach and completion of assigned tasks also give insight into the ability to work toward a specific goal.

Assessment through observation.   Skills such as speed, independence, and accuracy may be evaluated through observing and recording general and specific behavioral patterns—a process that is being accepted in most areas of education as a valuable assessment procedure, especially with young children or those who have numerous problems or impairments. For teachers, observing children on a one-to-one basis and also in groups is probably the simplest means of gathering information about present functioning. Teachers of visually handicapped children should be encouraged to use observation freely and consistently. To become a sophisticated observer may require time to learn to select appropriate situations for observation, significant behaviors and responses, and practical procedures for recording what is seen.

For example, children may be observed in free play in a variety of totally *unstructured* settings; or the environment and the materials available for use may be *semistructured* to limit to some extent the behaviors possible or to encourage certain desired responses; or the situation may be *structured* to require a specific type of task performance or interaction.

Whatever the setting or situation, knowing *what to observe* is critical. Each observer may be interested in assessing particular behaviors and consequently focus exclusively on those. Observing the following behaviors can provide pertinent information about visually handicapped children: (1) awareness of, and attention to, the surrounding environment and those within it, (2) seeking and exploratory patterns of movement, (3) use of the senses in moving and acquiring information, (4) use of language to elicit contact or to respond to encounters, (5) nature and variety of cues used for self-directive and independent actions, and (6) extent to which the child originates behavior or adapts to materials or to people. These few suggestions may stimulate teachers and others to develop their own ideas about what to observe.

Carefully recording the observations on checklists or scales can help estimate the developmental and functional status of children across affective, psychomotor, and cognitive dimensions. A profile plotted or drawn across all the behavioral domains gives the teacher a basis for determining some reasonable short-term objectives and for planning appropriate tasks or interactions to help children move toward their achievement.

Although observational evaluation may be the most desirable procedure for some children, others may profit by more extensive or standardized assessment techniques. The following model presents an ideal assessment technique, which presumes that all visually handicapped children will be available for evaluation prior to entering school. Whatever the age or level of the child when he enters an educational program, the assessment process should begin at the preschool level and progress sequentially as far as is appropriate. In addition, observational techniques should be incorporated whenever suitable.

Preschool Assessment

Medical information: Nature and severity of visual impairment and prognosis as to whether the condition is stable, operable, or deteriorating; prescriptions for lenses or optical aids and for what purposes they are to be used.

Family history and experience: A complete analysis of family attitudes and expectations in addition to the general characteristics. A home visit by a case worker, social worker, or teacher should be an integral part of this procedure.

Maxfield-Buchholz Social Maturity Scale: May be administered during home visit and verified by future observations.

Checklists or development scales: May be begun during home visit and completed on subsequent visits or contacts. These indicate physical, personal-social-emotional, and language development.

Counseling parents and suggestions for preschool learning experiences can be based on the lags or defects detected through the assessment procedures. Continued periodic evaluation is desirable throughout the first five or six years to ensure appropriate interventions to prepare children for beginning more formal academic learning when they enter school.

Primary and Elementary Assessment

Teacher observation and checklists: Teachers should record information derived from both informal and formal observation of movement behavior, use of hands in exploration, use of residual vision, and response to sound and auditory stimuli. Teacher-made checklists are valuable also for recording levels of development in personal skills, social skills, and other functional behaviors.

Achievements tests: To be used no earlier than second grade and probably not until third or fourth grade.

Roughness Discrimination Test: Blind only.

Tactual discrimination worksheets: Blind only.

Body Image Scale (Cratty and Sams, 1968).

Scale of Orientation and Mobility Skills (Lord, 1967).

Visual Efficiency Scale: Low vision and visually limited.

Nonlanguage Learning Test

Blind Learning Aptitude Test: Blind only.

Perkins-Binet and/or Wechsler Intelligence Scale for Children: Verbal portion only, and preferably after one or two years in school. The scores should be evaluated only as present functioning and not as predictors of potential.

Junior and Senior High School Assessment

Adolescent Emotional Factors Inventory

Haptic Intelligence Scale: Age sixteen and above.

Stanford-Kohs Block Design Test: Age sixteen and above.

Wechsler Adult Intelligence Scale: Age sixteen and above.

Scholastic Achievement Test

Interest inventories

Assessment and evaluation at the secondary level are valuable for counseling regarding the student's potential for advanced academic work or for specific vocational goals. Determining aptitude and interest in specific vocations is important as a basis for selecting training and could minimize the tendency to try to fit youth to a vocation rather than helping them identify the vocations for which they are suited. Continued assessment should be made of family attitudes, personal management skills, and the competencies necessary for independent living. The more information given young people, the greater the likelihood of their success in future life.

9

Paths Toward Independence

In the lives of most visually handicapped children, youth, and some adults, many conflicts seem to exist—between the goals of education and those of rehabilitation agencies, both of which may give too little consideration to the personal desires and needs of the individual. The prevailing assumption of most school programs is that their primary role is to see that each child develops to the maximum intellectually, often disregarding personal and vocational development. Much time and effort are invested in academic pursuits, even when the student's potential for independent living and functioning may be limited.

On the other hand, premature decisions to train for one specific occupational skill or vocation may pose an equally perplexing dilemma for the youth who leaves school and finds that no opportunities are available for him to practice his limited skills. Service delivery systems in rehabilitation for visually handicapped persons are geared almost exclusively to blinded adults who have already been a part of the work force or have previously established vocational or professional goals. They have only one major problem—loss of vision (OSTI, 1971).

Community and state agencies tend to provide a set of undifferentiated services defined by the agency itself and not necessarily related to the needs of the clients they serve. Educational programs and specialized schools have their own traditional, although not necessarily realistic, objectives for individual students or for career possibilities (Scott, 1969). Habilitation and rehabilitation begin at birth and continue until death, but so does education. Thus, conflicts between them are artificial and detrimental.

Perhaps educators need to define more clearly the long-range goals for each individual. Estimating possible performance in real life ten or fifteen years hence may determine the importance assigned to the number of arithmetic problems that were correctly solved today. For some youth, development in interpersonal relations or simply learning how to learn or to think and act independently or to achieve a sense of responsibility may be far more significant than grades or academic subject matter. Accumulating facts and acquiring an ability to verbalize about the world may delude the student (and sometimes teachers and parents as well) into thinking that such facilities are more important than being able to be self-directive and make realistic decisions about personal matters. Permitting visually handicapped youth to "graduate" from educational programs without ever having been given the experience of shopping for food, clothing, and other personal items makes a mockery of education.

Educators must learn a great deal more about the occupational, vocational, and career world in which the rehabilitation counselor functions. Counselors in agencies must learn more about educational and school philosophies, curriculum offerings, social and recreational opportunities, vocational programs, and the scope of mobility programs. The present gap between education and rehabilitation may be bridged if both were to consider a broader range of variables affecting all visually handicapped children and youth, some of which are discussed in the following pages.

Nature and Scope of Physical Impairments

In the past and to some degree at present, both education and rehabilitation have designed their programs for youth whose major or only recognized impairment was in the visual sense. Schools have thought primarily of congenital conditions, whereas rehabilitation has virtually ignored congenital impairments and directed their services toward the adventitiously impaired adult client (OSTI, 1971). A large proportion of students in schools are those like Carl and Lucy, who have conditions existing from birth; but a greater number of youth like Dora have degenerative conditions, or like Keith, suffer accidents during their school years. In addition, many children and youth have biological and physical impairments that affect several body organs and systems, creating multihandicaps (discussed in Chapter 5).

Some of the characteristic causal and sociological factors have a more marked influence on the social, personal, and emotional development of visually handicapped youth today than was true during the past hundred years. Severely visually handicapped children, youth, and adults have been detached or disengaged from the mainstream of society, at least to some degree, and despite a few exceptions, many have lived, learned, and participated on the periphery rather than in the center of family and community life (Rusalem, 1972). The medical cause of a condition and the general attitude of the family and school have done little to provide opportunity or encouragement for reality testing—that is, coping with the outside world without assistance.

Because a youth is visually handicapped is no reason to shield him from the normal stresses and failures that are part of life at all ages and stages of development. To be prevented from learning through failure, suffering the consequences of carelessness or poor planning, or competing with sighted peers denies a youth the very opportunities that enable him to achieve a sense of humanness and personhood and prepare him for the experience of life. Educators must focus more attention on the visually handicapped student's personality development, his attitudes toward self and others, and his mental health and interpersonal relationships.

Vocational and Economic Considerations

Career and vocational preparation are closely related to economic factors. If the federal and state governments were to invest funds for acquainting the visually handicapped with, and preparing them for, careers or vocations in which there is a predictable high probability of success, not only would society be required to spend less for habilitation *after* the school years, but there would also be greater productivity from goods, services, and taxes provided by congenitally visually handicapped persons. Independence or even partial independence at an earlier age would reduce the need for many of the economic expenditures associated with caring for the visually handicapped. Aside from the economic benefits, the human considerations are important. Knowing that one has skills that are economically valuable and that using those skills provides personal satisfaction can be motivations for increased independence.

Reports from rehabilitation teachers regarding the inability of some blind youths to carry a tray from a cafeteria line, to prepare a sandwich or a simple meal for themselves, or to manage their own money are no less than heartbreaking. One may wonder what good a high school diploma will do these young people when they have been deprived of the opportunity to learn how to live. A recent publication by Davidow, called *A Guide for Social Competency* (1974), would be an excellent textbook for visually handicapped junior and senior high school students. Practical learning experiences may be related more to achieving independence than to acquiring a particular knowledge or skill.

Developing realistic attitudes about the facts of visual handicaps is as much a part of vocational preparation for independence as is acquiring knowledge and skills. Medical costs may be great in some cases because of eye conditions; living expenses may be proportionately higher for personal services and travel expenses in some careers; reduced income is a regrettable but real possibility. Young adults need to understand and accept these facts, at least until some changes occur. Counseling courses and small-group "rap" sessions with visually handicapped adults who are currently pursuing vocations can be very informative, since evidence suggests that many young people who are visually handicapped are naïve about the responsibilities, the demands, and the stresses experienced in many occupations. Their knowledge about occupations and vocations is often limited in scope as well as depth. Providing opportunities for participating in simulated work experiences, for developing "mini" work stations, permitting students to work as occupational aides and in actual on-the-job training would be a tremendous benefit, since reading or hearing about what one does in a certain job may have little meaning if the action itself has never been performed. Cooperation between educational and rehabilitation agencies has the potential to be both economically and vocationally more productive than is the present system of separation. Many state and local agencies are moving toward a stronger coordination of activities among local schools, residential schools, and community or state rehabilitation agencies in providing career information, vocational education, and job training.

Alternative Educational Programming

Surveys and studies of visually handicapped young adults who have graduated from both local and residential school programs indicate that a high percentage are either overeducated and underemployed or show a great inconsistency in job stability far beyond that of the general population (Scholl, Bauman, and Crissey, 1969). It may be that visually handicapped youth have no philosophical understanding of work as an integral part of a full life. Work can be viewed in two ways: work as a goal and work as a process. Perhaps education should be seen as both a goal and a process. Without considering the process a major focus, attaining either work or education as a goal is unlikely. Any process is a continuum of skills, training, experiences, evaluation, and reevaluation directed toward both general and specific goals. To the present time, most school programs have been narrowly concerned with the goal of teaching academic subject matter. Rethinking the content of educational programs for the variable population of visually handicapped youth may be in order. Or, the time may have come to consider a constellation of school programs and vocational services in large cities or in states, each providing a different program and serving youth for specified goals. (A hypothetical model for a comprehensive state plan, from birth to economic and vocational independence, was presented in Chapter 7.)

Regardless of the process by which the objective of independence is realized, the learnings and skills—both academic and vocational—that must be part of the educational curriculum for visually handicapped youth have been established. All of these career skills bear a strong relationship to the personal, social, economic, and vocational factors discussed earlier in this chapter, and they presently comprise some portion of various residential programs around the country (Carroll and LaBarre, 1974; Clayton, 1971; Coker, 1974; Rossi and Marotta, 1974). Unfortunately, few public school programs have expanded much beyond the academic curriculum. Perhaps comprehensive programming in local schools is not feasible. If this is the case, the previous suggestion of state planning among many agencies has great validity. Whatever the approaches toward education and rehabilitation, all visually handicapped youth have the right to expect equal opportunity for preparation for a productive life. The outline below presents the primary components of a career educational program.

I. Personal, social, and everyday living skills to provide confidence, ease, and comfort in functioning, and independence in living arrangements.
    A. Knowledge and understanding of self as a person.
       1. Interests, capabilities, limitations.
       2. Attitudes about self and others.
       3. Personality characteristics and self-concept.
       4. Sexual identity, needs, and behaviors.
    B. Personal care and management.
       1. Eating, dressing, grooming.
       2. Selecting, purchasing, and caring for appropriate clothing.
       3. Skills in hair arrangement, tying ties, use of self-care tools.
    C. Social skills.
       1. Good manners and appropriate behaviors.
       2. Games and leisure-time activities.
       3. Interaction with others, especially sighted persons and those of the opposite sex.
    D. Home management.
       1. Selecting, purchasing, and preparing simple foods and meals.
       2. Use and manipulation of simple materials, utensils, and equipment.
       3. Simple mechanical repairs.
       4. Managing personal finances and budgets.
II. Realistic communication and business skills.
    A. Information gathering for study or for vocational preparation.
       1. Sources of available materials in all media.
       2. Selection and appropriate use of reading devices and equipment such as optical aids, listening equipment, Optacon, and others.
    B. Written communication.
       1. Braille labelling and organization of materials for efficiency.
       2. Typing skills for personal, vocational, and professional purposes.
       3. Formats for tax forms, bookkeeping, and so on.
    C. Computational and measurement skills.
       1. Selection and use of appropriate devices for home and occupational purposes.
       2. Inventory and recording accuracy.
III. Concept development, precane skills, and independent mobility.
    A. Orientation of self to objects and space.
       1. Functional understanding of vocabulary related to movement and spatial alignment.

      2. Knowledge and skill in movement of body.
      3. Spatial orientation to work area of in-reach space.
  B. Organization of work areas and equipment.
      1. Arrangement of tools, materials, and/or devices for efficient use in a variety of job stations.
      2. Skill in spatial location of needed objects and return to designated positions after use.
      3. Maintenance of orderly work area in numerous work stations.
  C. Exploration and movement in familiar and unfamiliar environments.
      1. Skill in exploration of work space, classrooms, and other indoor settings.
      2. Efficient movement between work settings and/or classrooms and building.
  D. Independent travel.
      1. Cane travel or use of guide dogs in school and neighborhood areas.
      2. Use of public transportation to and from school and/or job setting.
      3. Travel in suburban and city areas without assistance.
IV. Career, vocational, and/or technical occupations.
  A. Exploration of, and exposure to, appropriate careers, vocations, or technical occupations.
      1. Simulation of work experiences.
      2. Group discussions with successful visually handicapped persons working in various roles.
      3. Workshop, office, business, or professional work experience in community.
  B. Training in general work skills.
      1. Attitudes toward self and others in work settings.
      2. General work habits and skills common to many vocations.
      3. General safety and manipulative skills related to various settings, such as laboratory, business, workshop, and/or professional careers.
  C. Training in skills for specific vocations, occupations, or professional careers.
      1. Selection according to interest, predicted potential for success, personal and family considerations.
      2. Skill development in work stations, contract work, or in-school work experiences.
      3. Placement in on-the-job training sites with full responsibility in community.

To the extent that such a plan or portions of it are feasible, the educational program could be designed to provide individual and group counseling opportunities to support and supplement actual experiences. Additional or complementary academic courses could be selected to provide or strengthen knowledge in areas of deficiencies or observed weaknesses. As the trend toward year-round educational programs increases, quarters of intensive career preparation could become the responsibility of residential campuses, and quarters of concentrated academic work might be provided in public schools. All visually handicapped youth would be assigned to a program according to individual needs.

Programs of this nature might provide each young person leaving an educational program some knowledge of "where to go," "how to get there," and "what to expect along the way." Until such goals are achieved, educators may be inhibiting, rather than contributing to, independence in adulthood for visually handicapped youth as participating, contributing members of society.

10

Knowledge into Practice

What is actually known about learning in children and youth with visual handicaps is a controversial issue among philosophers, medical and optical specialists, and educators. The hope of reaching agreement is an illusion that often inhibits effectively implementing available knowledge into practice with students. With due respect to those whose ideas may differ from mine, in this chapter I shall present a short summary of the issues and trends I consider critical and suggest priorities for practical applications of what is presently known. Documentation for everything discussed here has already been presented. The reader should have no difficulty referring to other sections of the text for objective data, if desired.

Critical Issues Summarized

The first issue underlying all others is that of *definitions*. The reasons for using legal and medical designations of "blindness" may be valid for some purposes but have been found inadequate, inappropriate, and confusing when applied to children or when adopted as eligibility criteria for educational services. The word *blind* (regardless of such descriptive prefixes as "legally" or "medically") has the universal connotation of a lack of vision. In relation to learning and functioning during school years, the term *blind* should be used only when the impairment is so extensive that no usable vision is present. Strategies and interventions to facilitate learning and development are different from those for normally seeing children. Almost without exception, the special needs are similar for all blind children and may be furnished by parents, specialists, and teachers in a variety of settings.

Children and youth who are aware of, and respond to, light and other visual stimuli, but who demonstrate inconsistent visual behavioral characteristics, are less easily designated as a group. The nature and causes of the impairments may be quite different; the potential for visual development cannot be estimated accurately; and the clarity of what they see under different conditions is specific to each individual. The one quality they have in common may be their inability to see at distances of more than a few feet. Logically, they may be defined as having *low vision,* and for educational purposes, the planning and implementation of learning experiences for this group has some similarities as well as many differences. The developmental needs and functional expectancies for low-vision children will not be the same as those for blind children because of the attention to visual stimulation and the guidance required to make use of residual vision.

The largest proportion of children and youth with visual problems are those who have less severe impairments and are able to function visually, to some extent, in most situations. However, the impairments cannot be repaired or corrected to give clear, sharp near or distance vision under any conditions. In development, learning, and functioning, this group is *visually limited.* Parents, teachers, and others should be aware of the type of visual problem present and understand how the visual behavior will be affected.

Those whose characteristics fall within any of these three groups may be defined as *visually handicapped* in relation to educational needs. All of them will require adaptations in materials and media, teaching techniques, lighting conditions, and different programming arrangements beyond those necessary for children with normal vision. With appropriate identification and planning, the development and learning of visually handicapped children and youth can approximate the patterns found in all children, from slow to average to fast. Definitions and labelling should be for the purpose of permitting children to be included in, and not excluded from, the mainstream of life's activities.

A second issue is *recognizing the critical need for intervention immediately after birth* for all children with visual impairments. The time of highest priority for maximal development and future learning is during the child's first four or five years of life. For *blind* children and their parents, the first two years are the most critical period to minimize the emotional and physical isolation and to emphasize body movement and tactual exploration. Without the opportunity for developing attachment, knowledge, participation, and involvement with people and objects, the blind child's foundations for later learning and freedom of movement will remain incomplete.

The first two or three years are equally critical for *low-vision* children and their parents. Attention to visual stimulation at close range will enhance the rate and quality of visual development within the limits of the child's potential for useful vision, which in turn will help stimulate and accelerate psychomotor and cognitive development. Low-vision children may be unaware of what they can see and learn visually and begin to lag needlessly in their development, unless parents and teachers understand the limitations for spontaneous visual development.

Visually limited children whose impairments are identified early in life have a better chance to profit by optical or surgical intervention that might possibly permit more normal visual development. Even when conditions are not totally correctable, parents and teachers can be more sensitive to visual limitations and adjust environmental conditions to foster optimal learning experiences.

A third issue that is still perplexing is *recognizing and accepting the diversity of multi-impairments* among visually handicapped children. Whether there are actually greater numbers of visually handicapped children who have additional impairments today than there were in previous years has not been established. Possibly improved diagnostic and assessment procedures along with changing societal attitudes toward damaged children have called our attention to those who might at one time have been institutionalized as "hopeless." One fact is clear: A smaller portion of children in educational settings have only visual impairments. Long-term interdisciplinary evaluation is required to identify the myriad of interactive factors interfering with development, and predictions for future learning potential are tenuous at best. Individual prescriptive planning for each child appears to be the only productive approach. Time, money, a range of service-delivery systems, and a cadre of interdisciplinary personnel are needed to implement effective programs for this challenging group of children.

The fourth issue—the critical factors relating to *tactual, auditory, and visual learning*—is of major educational importance. Psychological and educational research have revealed information about human learning and perceptual-cognitive processing of sensory information that we have just begun to translate and apply to visually handicapped children and youth. A sequence of concrete readiness experiences designed for primary and alternative learning senses will enable children to interpret the more abstract symbols of letter and word forms and sounds. Facilitating the development of ear-hand and hand-brain coordination is essential for all children with visual problems. The information received from the same object is different when the perceiver uses the tactual, auditory, or visual sense. It follows that the responses of visually handicapped children may differ from those of normally sighted children, depending on the sense(s) used in learning.

Educational Trends

A definite trend toward *expanded educational programming and greater use of technology* has emerged in recent years. Programs for visually handicapped children and youth are now found in local public schools, community agencies, early childhood centers, as well as in the traditional state or private residential schools. Electronic devices have been developed as alternatives to sensory information gathering, and production of braille and recorded material has become more efficient through the use of electronic equipment. Several states are in the process of developing statewide service-delivery systems, which provide for organized and coordinated programs across all state agencies serving visually handicapped children and youth. Such plans will ensure appropriate services to all visually handicapped children and their parents and will minimize the possibility of fragmentation or gaps between agencies and programs. We know that continuity between diagnosis, evaluation, intervention, and follow-up can enhance the child's development and learning. The hope that such continuity could become a reality through comprehensive state programs under the direction of one responsible administrator is an exciting prospect.

A long-awaited trend in assessment and evaluation is placing the emphasis on *individual learning and functioning characteristics.* Research studies stress the uniqueness of individual performance within the groups, even when data are analyzed according to group samples. Distinctions are now being made between those who are totally blind and those who have useful residual vision, in addition to distinguishing among congenital impairments, those occurring in the first three or four years of life, and those occurring after the preschool years. Making such distinctions permits the accumulation of more precise and reliable data from which to design and modify intervention strategies and to create new learning approaches. Still lacking but of pressing concern are criteria to use as accurate predictors of developmental and learning potential. Refinement in theoretical rationale and investigative techniques for experimental research is providing more valid data. Translating the growing body of knowledge into educational practice with visually handicapped children and youth is the present objective.

Perhaps a more hopeful than real trend is incorporating into the educational curriculum *vocational and career preparation,* rather than considering this a rehabilitative process after school years. Although a few educators are giving attention to vocational and career preparation as part of the curriculum, we have only begun to accept the notion that preparation for living means the ability to be productive, to find joy and satisfaction in independence, and to experience the dignity of feeling competent and valuable.

The Challenge

New discoveries about the development and learning of visually handicapped children are occurring rapidly. Unfortunately, educational practices do not necessarily employ all available knowledge. Some teachers may not have access to new ideas or may have difficulty translating them into practice. More probably, the lag in putting new knowledge into practice arises from a reluctance to question traditional attitudes and methods or from a lack of courage to take the risks implied in making dynamic and innovative changes.

The visually handicapped children and youth in our educational programs deserve educational activities appropriate to their present level of functioning and designed to help them move, step-by-step, up the ladder of independence to a life of freedom and dignity. Teachers could be the leaders in achieving this goal, but will they?

References

Abel, G. L. Problems and trends in the education of blind children and youth. In G. L. Abel, ed., *Concerning the education of blind children.* New York: American Foundation for the Blind, 1959, pp. 79–101.

Arnheim, R. *Visual thinking.* London: Faber & Faber, 1969.

Ashcroft, S. C. Delineating the possible for the multi-handicapped child with visual impairment. *International Journal for the Education of the Blind,* 1966, 16, 52–55.

Ashcroft, S. C.; Halliday, C.; and Barraga, N. C. *Study II: Effects of experimental teaching on the visual behavior of children educated as though they had no vision.* Nashville, Tenn.: George Peabody College for Teachers, 1965.

Barraga, N. C. *Increased visual behavior in low vision children.* New York: American Foundation for the Blind, 1964.

————. Utilization of sensory-perceptual abilities. In B. Lowenfeld, ed., *The visually handicapped child in school.* New York: John Day, 1973, pp. 117–54.

————, ed. *Teacher's guide for development of visual learning abilities and utilization of low vision.* Louisville, Ky.: American Printing House for the Blind, 1970.

————, ed. *Visual Efficiency Scale.* Louisville, Ky.: American Printing House for the Blind, 1970.

Barraga, N. C.; Dorward, B.; and Ford, P. *Aids for teaching basic concepts of sensory development.* Louisville, Ky.: American Printing House for the Blind, 1973.

Bateman, B. Psychological evaluation of blind children. *New Outlook for the Blind,* 1965, 59, 193–97.

Bateman, B., and Weatherall, J. L. Some educational characteristics of partially seeing children. *International Journal for the Education of the Blind,* 1967, 17, 33–40.

Bauman, M. K. Psychological and educational assessment. In B. Lowenfeld, ed., *The visually handicapped child in school.* New York: John Day, 1973, pp. 93–115.

Bauman, M. K.; Platt, H.; and Strauss, S. A measure of personality for blind adolescents. *International Journal for the Education of the Blind,* 1963, 13(1), 7–12.

Best, J. T., and Winn, R. J. A place to go in Texas. *International Journal for the Education of the Blind*, 1968, 18, 2–9.

Birch, J. W.; Tisdall, W. J.; Peabody, R.; and Sterrett, R. School achievement and effect of type size on reading in visually handicapped children. *Cooperative Research Project No. 1766, U.S. Office of Education*. Pittsburgh: Univ. of Pittsburgh Press, 1966.

Bishop, V. E. *Teaching the visually limited child*. Springfield, Ill.: Charles C Thomas, 1971.

Bliss, J. C., and Moore, M. W. The Optacon reading system. *Education of the Visually Handicapped*, 1974, 6, 98–102.

Boldt, W. The development of scientific thinking in blind children and adolescents. *Education of the Visually Handicapped*, 1969, 1, 5–11.

Brothers, R. J. Aural study systems for the visually handicapped. *Education of the Visually Handicapped*, 1971, 3, 65–70.

————. Arithmetic computation by the blind: A look at current achievements. *Education of the Visually Handicapped*, 1972, 4, 1–8.

Bruner, J. S. *Toward a theory of instruction*. New York: Norton, 1966.

Buktenica, N. A. *Visual learning*. San Raphael, Calif.: Dimension, 1968.

Bullard, B., and Barraga, N. C. Subtests of evaluative instruments applicable for use with pre-school visually handicapped children. *Education of the Visually Handicapped*, 1971, 3, 116–22.

Calhoun, R. C.; Lutz, G. W.; and Knab, K. *San Diego Optacon project—1971–1972*. San Diego, Calif.: San Diego Unified School District, 1972.

Carroll, L. R., and LeBarre, A. H. A cooperative vocational guidance course for visually impaired students-clients. *New Outlook for the Blind*, 1974, 68, 163–69.

Chase, J. B. Evaluation of blind and severely visually impaired persons. In M. D. Graham, ed., *Science and blindness: Retrospective and prospective*. New York: American Foundation for the Blind, 1972.

Clayton, I. P. An expanded program in prevocational education at The Maryland School for the Blind. *Education of the Visually Handicapped*, 1971, 3, 80–81.

Coker, D. G. The development of a vocational program in a residential school for the visually handicapped. *New Outlook for the Blind*, 1974, 68, 25–28.

Coveny, T. E. A new test for the visually handicapped: Preliminary analysis of the reliability and validity of the Perkins-Binet. *Education of the Visually Handicapped*, 1972, 4, 97–101.

Cratty, B. J., and Sams, T. *Body image of blind children*. New York: American Foundation for the Blind, 1968.

————. *Movement and spatial awareness in blind children and youth*. Springfield, Ill.: Charles C Thomas, 1971.

Davidow, M. E. *A guide for social competency*. Louisville, Ky.: American Printing House for the Blind, 1974.

Davis, C. J. New developments in the intelligence testing of blind children. In *Proceedings of the conference on new approaches to the evaluation of blind persons.* New York: American Foundation for the Blind, 1970.

Dauterman, W. L.; Shapiro, B.; and Suinn, R. M. Performance tests of intelligence for the blind reviewed. *International Journal for the Education of the Blind,* 1967, 17, 8–16.

Dickman, I. R. *Sex education and family life for visually handicapped children and youth: A resource guide.* New York: American Foundation for the Blind, 1972.

Eakin, W. M.; Pratt, R. J.; and McFarland, F. *Type-size research for the partially seeing child.* Pittsburgh: Stanwix House, 1961.

Enis, C. A., and Cataruzolo, M. Sex education in the residential school for the blind. *Education of the Visually Handicapped,* 1972, 4, 61–64.

Erikson, E. H. Play and actuality. In M. W. Piers, ed., *Play and development.* New York: Norton, 1972, pp. 127–67.

Faye, E. E. *The low vision patient.* New York: Grune & Stratton, 1970.

Fieandt, K. *The world of perception.* Homewood, Ill.: Dorsey Press, 1966.

Fonda, G. An evaluation of large type. *New Outlook for the Blind,* 1966, 60, 296–98.

Foulke, E. Non-visual communication. *International Journal for the Education of the Blind,* 1968, 18, 77–78.

_____. Non-visual communication: Reading by listening. *Education of the Visually Handicapped,* 1969, 1, 79–81.

Fraiberg, S.; Smith, M.; and Adelson, E. An educational program for blind infants. *Journal of Special Education,* 1969, 3, 121–39.

Fraiberg, S., and Adelson, E. Self-representation in language and play: Observations of blind children. *Psychoanalytic Quarterly,* 1973, 42, 539–62.

Furth, H. G. *Piaget and knowledge.* Englewood Cliffs, N.J.: Prentice-Hall, 1969.

Goldish, L. H. *Teaching aids for the visually handicapped.* Watertown, Mass.: Perkins School for the Blind, 1968.

Gore, G. V. A comparison of two methods of speeded speech. *Education of the Visually Handicapped,* 1969, 1, 69–76.

Graham, M. D. *Multiply-impaired blind children: A national problem.* New York: American Foundation for the Blind, 1968.

Gruber, K. F., and Moor, P. M., eds. *No place to go.* New York: American Foundation for the Blind, 1963.

Halliday, C. *The visually impaired child—growth, learning, development—infancy to school age.* Louisville, Ky.: American Printing House for the Blind, 1970.

Hammill, B., and Crandell, J. N. Implications of tactile-kinesthetic ability in visually handicapped children. *Education of the Visually Handicapped,* 1969, 1, 65–69.

Hapeman, L. B. Developmental concepts of blind children between the ages of three and six as they relate to orientation and mobility. *International Journal for the Education of the Blind,* 1967, 17, 41–48.

Hardy, R. E. A study of manifest anxiety among blind residential school students. *New Outlook for the Blind,* 1968, 62, 173–80.

Harley, R., and Spollen, J. A study of the reliability and validity of the Visual Efficiency Scale with low vision children. *Education of the Visually Handicapped,* 1973, 5, 110–14.

Harley, R.; Spollen, J.; and Long, S. A study of the reliability and validity of the Visual Efficiency Scale with preschool children. *Education of the Visually Handicapped,* 1973, 5, 38–42.

Hayes, S. P. *Contributions to a psychology of blindness.* New York: American Foundation for the Blind, 1952.

Hebb, D. O. *The organization of behavior.* New York: John Wiley, 1949.

Henderson, F. Communication skills. In B. Lowenfeld, ed., *The visually handicapped child in school.* New York: John Day, 1973, pp. 185–219.

Higgins, L. C. *Classification in congenitally blind children.* New York: American Foundation for the Blind, 1973.

Hill, E. W. The formation of concepts in body position in space. *Education of the Visually Handicapped,* 1970, 2, 112–15.

Holmes, R. V. The planning and implementation of a sex education program for visually handicapped children in a residential setting. *New Outlook for the Blind,* 1974, 68, 219–25.

Hull, W. A., and McCarthy, C. G. Supplementary programs for preschool visually handicapped children. *Education of the Visually Handicapped,* 1973, 5, 97–104.

Hunt, J. M. *Intelligence and experience.* New York: Ronald Press, 1961.

Jones, J. W. *Blind children—degree of vision, mode of reading.* Washington, D.C.: U.S. Government Printing Office, 1961.

Jones, J. W., and Collins, A. T. *Educational programs for visually handicapped children.* Washington, D.C.: U.S. Government Printing Office, 1966.

Juurmaa, J. *Ability structure and loss of vision.* New York: American Foundation for the Blind, 1967.

Kempton, W. *A teacher's guide to sex education for persons with learning disabilities.* Belmont, Calif.: Duxbury Press, Wadsworth Publishing, 1975.

Keogh, B. K. Perceptual and cognitive styles: Implication for special education. *First Review of Special Education,* 1973, 83–109.

Kidwell, A. M., and Greer, T. S. *Sight, perception, and the nonvisual experience.* New York: American Foundation for the Blind, 1973.

Knight, J. J. Mannerisms in the congenitally blind child. *New Outlook for the Blind,* 1972, 66, 297–302.

Kratz, L. E. *Movement without sight.* Palo Alto, Calif.: Peek, 1973.

Lewis, M. Teaching arithmetic computation skills. *Education of the Visually Handicapped,* 1970, 2, 66–72.

Linville, J. G., and Bliss, J. C. *A direct translation reading aid for the blind.* Stanford, Calif.: Stanford Electronics Laboratories, 1965. (Report SEL–65–055, TR No. 4819–1.)

Lord, F. E. *Preliminary standardization of a scale of orientation and mobility skills of young blind children. Final report.* Los Angeles: California State College, 1967. (Grant No. OEG–4–7–062464, Proj. No. 6–2464.)

Lowenfeld, B. Multihandicapped blind and deaf-blind children in California. *Research Bulletin No. 19.* New York: American Foundation for the Blind, 1969, pp. 1–72.

_____. History of the education of visually handicapped children. In B. Lowenfeld, ed., *The visually handicapped child in school.* New York: John Day, 1973, pp. 1–25.

Lydon, W. T., and McGraw, M. L. *Concept development for visually handicapped children.* New York: American Foundation for the Blind, 1973.

McLaughlin, W. J. Reading attainment of blind and partially sighted children: A comparative study. *The Teacher of the Blind,* 1974, 62, 98–106.

Maxfield, K. E., and Buchholz, S. *A social maturity scale for blind preschool children.* New York: American Foundation for the Blind, 1957.

Montessori, M. *The discovery of the child.* New York: Ballantine, 1967.

Moore, M. W. *Professional preparation of teachers of reading with the Optacon.* Pittsburgh: University of Pittsburgh Press, 1973.

Morris, J. E. The 1973 Stanford Achievement Test Series as adapted for use by the visually handicapped. *Education of the Visually Handicapped,* 1974, 6, 33–40.

Murphy, L. B. Infants' play and cognitive development. In M. W. Piers, ed., *Play and development.* New York: Norton, 1972, pp. 119–26.

Napier, G. D. Special subject adjustments and skill. In B. Lowenfeld, ed., *The visually handicapped child in school.* New York: John Day, 1973, pp. 221–77.

Newland, T. E. The Blind Learning Aptitude Test. In *Conference on research on braille.* New York: American Foundation for the Blind, 1961.

Nolan, C. Y. Readability of large types—A study of type sizes and type styles. *International Journal for the Education of the Blind,* 1959, 9, 41–44.

_____. *Reading and listening in learning by the blind: Progress report.* Louisville, Ky.: American Printing House for the Blind, 1966.

Nolan, C. Y., and Kederis, C. J. *Perceptual factors in braille word recognition.* New York: American Foundation for the Blind, 1969.

Nolan, C. Y., and Morris, J. E. Development and validation of the Roughness Discrimination Test. *International Journal for the Education of the Blind,* 1965, 15, 1–6.

_____. *Aural study systems for the visually handicapped. Final Report, Project No. 8–0046.* Washington, D.C.: Dept. of HEW, 1973.

O'Brien, R. The integrated resource room for visually impaired children. *New Outlook for the Blind,* 1973, 67, 363–68.

Organization for Social and Technical Innovation. *Blindness and services to the blind in the United States.* Cambridge, Mass.: OSTI Press, 1971.

Piaget, J. *The psychology of intelligence.* Totowa, N.J.: Littlefield, Adams, 1966.

———. *Science of education and the psychology of the child.* New York: Orion Press, 1970.

———. *The child and reality.* New York: Grossman, 1973.

Rex, E. J. A study of basal readers and experimental supplementary instructional materials for teaching primary reading in braille. *Education of the Visually Handicapped,* 1970, 2, 97–107.

Rogow, S. M. Speech development and the blind multi-impaired child. *Education of the Visually Handicapped,* 1973, 4, 105–9.

Rossi, P., and Marotta, M. Breaking blind stereotypes through vocational placements. *New Outlook for the Blind,* 1974, 68, 29–32.

Rusalem, H. *Coping with the unseen environment.* New York: Teacher's College Press, 1972.

Scholl, G. T. The psychosocial effect of blindness: Implications for program planning in sex education. *New Outlook for the Blind,* 1974, 68, 201–9.

Scholl, G. T.; Bauman, M. K.; and Crissey, M. S. *A study of the vocational success of groups of the visually handicapped. Final report.* Washington, D.C.: Social and Rehabilitation Service Grant No. RD–2554–S, 1969.

Scott, R. A. *The making of blind men.* New York: Russell Sage, 1969.

Shurrager, H. C., and Shurrager, P. S. *Manual for the Haptic Intelligence Scale for adult blind.* Chicago: Psychology Research, 1964.

Simon, J. D., A course in spoken communications for high school students who are visually handicapped. *Education of the Visually Handicapped,* 1974, 6, 41–43.

Simpkins, K. An auditory training program from kindergarten through third grade. *Education of the Visually Handicapped,* 1971, 3, 70–73.

Stephens, B. Cognitive processes in the visually impaired. *Education of the Visually Handicapped,* 1972, 4, 106–11.

Streitfeld, J. W., and Avery, C. D. The WAIS and HIS tests as predictors of academic achievement in a residential school for the blind. *International Journal for the Education of the Blind,* 1968, 18, 73–77.

Suinn, R. M., and Dauterman, W. L. *Manual for the Stanford-Kohs Block Design Test for the blind.* Washington, D.C.: Vocational Rehabilitation Administration, 1966.

Suterko, S. Life adjustment. In B. Lowenfeld, ed., *The visually handicapped child in school.* New York: John Day, 1973, pp. 279–317.

Sykes, K. C. A comparison of the effectiveness of standard print and large print in facilitating the reading skills of visually impaired students. *Education of the Visually Handicapped,* 1971, 3, 97–105.

————. Print reading for visually handicapped children. *Education of the Visually Handicapped,* 1972, 4, 71–75.

Tait, P., ed. *Teacher's guide to listening education.* Philadelphia: Temple University Press, 1973.

Talkington, L. W. An exploratory program for blind-retarded. *Education of the Visually Handicapped,* 1972, 2, 33–35.

Taylor, J. L. Educational programs. In B. Lowenfeld, ed., *The visually handicapped child in school.* New York: John Day, 1973, pp. 155–84.

Tillman, M. H. The performance of blind and sighted children on the Wechsler Intelligence Scale for Children. *International Journal for the Education of the Blind,* 1967, 16, 106–12.

Tobin, M. J. Conservation of substance in the blind and partially sighted. *British Journal of Educational Psychology,* 1972, 42, 192–97.

Tuttle, D. W. A comparison of three reading media for the blind. *Education of the Visually Handicapped,* 1972, 4, 40–44.

Valvo, A. *Sight restoration after long-term blindness: The problems and behavior patterns of visual rehabilitation.* New York: American Foundation for the Blind, 1971.

van'T. Hooft, F., and Heslinga, K. Sex education of blind-born children. *New Outlook for the Blind,* 1968, 62, 15–21.

Van Weelden, J. *On being blind.* Amsterdam: Netherlands Society for the Blind, 1967.

Warren, D. H. Early vs. late vision: The role of early vision in spatial reference systems. *New Outlook for the Blind,* 1974, 68, 157–62.

Weber, L. *The English infant school and informal education.* Englewood Cliffs, N.J.: Prentice-Hall, 1971.

Weiner, B. B. A new outlook on assessment. *New Outlook for the Blind,* 1967, 61, 73–78.

Witkin, H. A.; Oltman, C. K.; Chase, J. B.; and Freedman, F. Cognitive patterning in the blind. In J. Hellmuth, ed., *Cognitive studies—Deficits in cognition.* New York: Brunner/Mazel, 1971, pp. 16–46.

Wolf, J. M. *The blind child with concomitant disabilities.* New York: American Foundation for the Blind, 1967.

Index